D1602530

Kylo-Patrick R. Hart, PhD

The AIDS Movie
Representing a Pandemic in Film and Television

*Pre-publication
REVIEWS,
COMMENTARIES,
EVALUATIONS . . .*

"**W**ith this landmark analysis, Kylo-Patrick Hart offers readers the definitive work on representations of HIV/AIDS contained in American movies over the past two decades. Incorporating rich thinking and impressive analytical insights, Hart's discussion provides an intelligent overview of the negative social and ideological repercussions resulting from the dramatic over-reliance by filmmakers on portraying AIDS primarily as a disease of 'deviants' and a plague of the city. It focuses attention on eye-opening, at times startling issues pertaining to modern-day conceptions of social power, status, and 'otherness.'

This book explores a remarkably noteworthy body of films long overlooked by media studies scholars. In addition to defining and proposing criteria for identifying an 'AIDS movie,' it contains an impressive list of source materials and a comprehensive list of American movies that represent HIV/AIDS. Hart's ultimate creation is destined to remain an important theoretical and informational resource for many years to come. It is satisfying reading for anyone with a serious interest in film studies, television studies, cultural studies, sociology, gay and lesbian studies, or related fields."

Dr. Richard Allen
*Associate Professor
of Communication Studies,
University of Michigan,
Ann Arbor*

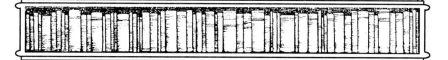

"Kylo-Patrick Hart's *The AIDS Movie: Representing a Pandemic in Film and Television* is an extremely well-written exploration of this film genre. It nicely places the AIDS movie within the context of cinematic history, and provides clear and economical sketches of these films that make the text accessible even to those who haven't seen them.

The text is also full of useful information about the history of the pandemic—including how it was initially treated by the media, what populations are showing increased levels of AIDS infection, etc. The fourth chapter, on the ways in which gay men are presented as the main victims of AIDS, is particularly informative as it also seeks to capture the way homosexuality has been represented in and of itself by the media.

The cultural studies approach that Hart takes allows him to capture the potential power of the AIDS movie in its ability to affect social change. Hart argues that these films have the ability to represent AIDS as a threat to all of us, although they have so far represented AIDS as a disease likely only to affect gay men. Hence, the suggestion that these films have been socially irresponsible comes through in his analysis of the genre,

as well as does the idea that they could do so much more to educate and to prevent the spread of this deadly disease. Its political message is, however, a subtle one, and is, as a result, that much more effective."

Marla Weitzman, PhD
Associate Professor of English,
University of Virginia's
College at Wise

"In *The AIDS Movie*, Hart tackles the difficult task of defining a new genre, beginning by tracing the development of the AIDS pandemic as well as the AIDS narrative, and then carefully placing the AIDS movie among established genres such as melodrama and science fiction. With a strong grounding in film and genre theory as well as the cultural theories of representation, Hart details the AIDS movies' contribution to the social construction of AIDS, and the danger of continuing to represent AIDS as a 'gay man's' disease.

Hart clearly links the lack of progress in expanding film and television representations of AIDS to risks in the real world, where individuals continue to delude themselves that they are protected by their 'normalcy,' despite the changing nature of the infection rate for the general population.

Hart's book serves as evidence that cultural studies can be conducted with academic rigor and still be readable. His careful attention to detail in examining these films, his firm grasp of theoretical complexities, and his evenhanded treatment of the topic make this book a model for future scholarship in the field."

Elizabeth C. Powers
Chair,
Mass Communication Program,
University of Charleston,
West Virginia

The Haworth Press, Inc.

The AIDS Movie
Representing a Pandemic
in Film and Television

The AIDS Movie
Representing a Pandemic in Film and Television

Kylo-Patrick R. Hart, PhD

The Haworth Press®
New York • London • Oxford

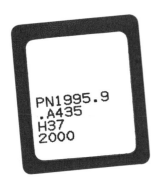

© 2000 by The Haworth Press, Inc. All rights reserved. No part of this work may be reproduced or utilized in any form or by any means, electronic or mechanical, including photocopying, microfilm, and recording, or by any information storage and retrieval system, without permission in writing from the publisher. Printed in the United States of America.

The Haworth Press, Inc., 10 Alice Street, Binghamton, NY 13904-1580

Cover design by Jennifer M. Gaska.

Library of Congress Cataloging-in-Publication Data

Hart, Kylo-Patrick R.
    The AIDS movie : representing a pandemic in film and television / Kylo-Patrick R. Hart.
        p.   cm.
    Includes bibliographical references and index.
    ISBN 0-7890-1107-7 (hard : alk. paper)—ISBN 0-7890-1108-5 (soft : alk. paper) 1. AIDS (Disease) in motion pictures. I. Title.

PN1995.9.A435 H37 2000
791.43'656—dc21
                                                 00-038879

For Joseph, Dorothy, Melissa, and Apollo

ABOUT THE AUTHOR

Kylo-Patrick Hart, PhD, is Assistant Professor of Mass Communication at the University of Virginia's College at Wise. He regularly teaches courses in mass communication; persuasion; film and television history, theory, and criticism; and cultural studies.

Dr. Hart's research interests include media representations of gay men and people with AIDS, cinematic spectatorship, and the impact of textual and visual messages on identity formation and public opinion.

Dr. Hart is an enthusiastic member of various academic associations, including the American Men's Studies Association, the Popular Culture Association, and the Society for Cinema Studies. His various writings on media representation have appeared in academic journals, including *The Journal of Men's Studies* and *Popular Culture Review,* and in the edited essay collection "Bang Bang, Shoot Shoot: Essays on Guns and Popular Culture."

CONTENTS

Preface

In the fall of 1996, at a meeting with Ross Chambers (author of *Facing It: AIDS Diaries and the Death of the Author*), I expressed my enthusiasm that the popular FOX television series *Beverly Hills 90210* had decided—after six full seasons on the air—to finally represent AIDS as an important social concern in one of its upcoming story lines. From the moment the series premiered, during the 1990 to 1991 television season, its producers and writers had made it a primary goal to regularly create episodes dealing candidly with contemporary social issues and concerns, ranging in topic from substance abuse by teens and young adults to homelessness, urban violence, and depression. Although character Kelly Taylor (played by Jennie Garth) informed others about the importance of using condoms and engaging in safer sexual practices during the show's first season, the absence of a true AIDS story line stood out as a glaring oversight by the end of its sixth season, especially given the regularity with which characters on the show found themselves involved in very casual sexual encounters.

The AIDS story line on *90210* consisted of nearly two dozen scenes, interspersed among various other story lines, during a consecutive three-week run in September 1996, near the start of the show's seventh season. The demographics of Americans being diagnosed with HIV/AIDS had, by then, undergone a dramatic change, as compared with those at the onset of the pandemic in the early 1980s (e.g., by the fall of 1996, transmission rates among gay men had fallen significantly, whereas those among heterosexual women, adolescents, and minority group members were reaching new heights annually). Knowing from viewer data that the majority of *90210* viewers in 1996 were women between the ages of eighteen and thirty-four, I had high hopes that the representation of AIDS on this show would be impressive, nonstereotypical, and somewhat on the cutting edge. Certainly, well into the second decade of AIDS, prime-time television had already offered more than its fill of stereotypical AIDS story lines, featuring little other than gay white males as their central AIDS characters. To my dismay, however, *90210* jumped on the prime-time bandwagon and featured a gay white male character named Jimmy as its central character with AIDS, one who was efficiently killed off after just three weeks and was not mentioned again in the weeks and months that followed.

Why had the producers and writers of *90210* chosen not to offer an alternate representation of AIDS, especially in an era when AIDS had become a leading cause of death among young Americans of all sexual orientations? Why had these individuals chosen to ignore the changing demographics of the AIDS pandemic by failing to create a story line that would be of greater relevance to their primary viewers, as evident from their own viewer demographics? Why had they resorted to prime-time television's standard "us" (uninfected "innocents") versus "them" (HIV- and AIDS-infected gay men who "threaten" the rest of society) plot development? These questions and related others haunted me for several weeks.

Findings from a series of focus groups I conducted at the University of Michigan with regular viewers of the series revealed that many others were as disappointed with this representation as I was. As one participant offered in an open-ended, written assessment of this representation, "I think it would have been better if Jimmy wasn't gay, because that might go against the [goal] of showing that this is a disease that anyone can get." Others explained, "The stereotyping of the gay guy with AIDS didn't really show us the reality of AIDS today" and "Jimmy was the stereotypical gay man with AIDS; it didn't 'hit home' that hard." In the end, the representation of AIDS on *Beverly Hills 90210* seemed more like something straight out of 1986, rather than 1996. (For a more complete analysis of the AIDS story line on *90210,* please see Kylo-Patrick R. Hart, "Retrograde Representation: The Lone Gay White Male Dying of AIDS on *Beverly Hills 90210," The Journal of Men's Studies,* Volume 7, Issue 2, Winter 1999, pp. 201-213).

Having been trained as a film scholar, my thoughts next drifted naturally to the representation of HIV/AIDS in American movies. The ones that sprung immediately to mind—*An Early Frost* (1985), *The*

Living End (1992), *Philadelphia* (1993), *It's My Party* (1996)—
appeared to offer little variation from the typical representation of
the gay white male dying of AIDS. As such, these offerings, similar
to the AIDS episodes of *Beverly Hills 90210,* failed to adequately
serve the needs of a wide range of audience members by ignoring
the changing demographics of the AIDS pandemic and reinforcing
the stigma associated with homosexuality in American society, as
well as the perception of AIDS as a disease perpetuated almost
exclusively by gay men, among other undesirable social outcomes.

Armed with extensive knowledge of the sociopsychological literature on stereotyping and prejudice, social stigma, and attitude
formation and change, and convinced that alternative representations of HIV/AIDS in American movies must have been produced
during the first two decades of the AIDS pandemic, I devoted the
next three years of my life to locating and analyzing as many
representations of AIDS in American movies as I could find. The
results of my exploration make up the chapters of this book. To the
best of my knowledge, this work represents the most comprehensive study of the cultural phenomenon of American movies about
AIDS that has yet been attempted. I hope this book will force
readers to reconsider and more fully challenge the pervasive nature
of ideology and social constructions in our understanding of AIDS
and people with AIDS, and that it will guide the creators of influential media messages in producing more effective representations of
HIV/AIDS that can help stem the tide of the AIDS pandemic as we
enter its third decade and (if necessary) beyond.

Kylo-Patrick R. Hart

Acknowledgments

Thank you, thank you, thank you to the many devoted mentors, teachers, researchers, colleagues, family members, and friends, past and present, who have, knowingly or unknowingly, contributed invaluably to the completion of this project, most notably, Richard Allen, José Arraguin, Richard Benjamin, Rebecca Bickley, Thomas Buhr, Karen Burke, Cindy Cantrell, Gregory Caybut, Diane Cerne, Ross Chambers, Donna Clapp, Loretta Coposky, Kaye Day, Tangela Diggs, Heidi Dvorak, Janet Fulk, Michelle Givertz, Patricia Gonzalez, Kristen Harrison, Apollo Hart, Ronald Heise, Steve Johnson, Victoria Johnson, Dorothy Kato, Joseph Kato, Melissa Kato, Gary Keck, Alix Andrea Kneifel, Ira Konigsberg, Leila Kramer, Kellie Lee, Debra Lewis, David Marc, Joan Marty, Lisa McLaughlin, Andrea Mullarkey, Sheila Murphy, Theresa Norgard, Hayg Oshagan, Brian Patrick, Elizabeth Powers, Austin Ranney, Willard Rodgers, Timothy "Buck" Roggeman, Ruth Seymour, Lisa Eva Siegler, Todd Smilovitz, Charles Stallman, Kathy Terrazas, Rachel Tighe, Kenneth Tiller, Laura Wackwitz, Marla Weitzman, Patricia Willis, S. Brandon Wu, and Amit Zohar.

Chapter 1

Conceptualizing the AIDS Movie
and Its Study

Dedicated to raising funds and awareness to combat the on-slaught of HIV and AIDS, the Red Hot Organization, in 1994, released an hour-long videocassette containing music videos and short films about AIDS by alternative music artists. It was designed to educate teenagers and young adults about the hazards associated with HIV/AIDS and to encourage safer sexual practices. The lyrics of one of the most intriguing and professionally executed offerings from that collection—the music video for the song "Take a Walk," by the band Urge Overkill—encourage (presumably uninfected) listeners to confront their feelings about people with AIDS and to see past all the stereotypes and fear, to start caring about these worthy individuals as if they were healthy because, fundamentally, they are no different from anyone else. The visual images accompa-nying those lyrics, however, convey quite a different message.

The visuals for "Take a Walk" offer glimpses of individuals in the advanced stages of AIDS. The video opens with two brief scenes of a Caucasian man lying solemnly on his (death)bed, ac-companied by lyrics explaining how the man no longer strives to survive because only alcoholic beverages (rather than individuals with AIDS) improve with age. These stark images and words set the tone for the remainder of the video—there is no hope here; death is inevitable. In rapid succession, the viewer is introduced to a second Caucasian man, now visibly wasting away, who holds a photograph of his face from healthier days gone by beside its current emaciated counterpart. Then comes a shot of a large African woman in a wheelchair, who stares lifelessly toward the heavens. This image is followed immediately by cutting to a third Caucasian man, outdoors and sobbing in his wheelchair, who covers his eyes as a latex-glove-covered hand reaches toward him. Next, the camera zooms in on the face of a fourth Caucasian man, whose gaunt features reveal the extent to which he has been ravaged by the disease. A bit later, the viewer encounters a mustached Hispanic man, who is being shaved and sponge-bathed by a glove-clad nurse. All of these individuals appear to be in their late twenties to midthirties. They make up the main characters of the video who return in later scenes, the infected individuals with whom the viewer is expected to identify.

As the music video proceeds, it becomes clear through the visual imagery that one of these individuals is dying because she comes from the AIDS-ravaged continent of Africa, and another is dying because he injected drugs through hypodermic needles shared with infected others. As for the rest, they seem to be dying primarily because they are gay men, with an early death portrayed as the virtually inevitable outcome of life in the gay community. For all six characters in the video, embracing death is their only option. After presenting a few momentary glimpses of happier, more optimistic times gone by in the middle of the video—two nude men smiling and embracing, spring flowers in full bloom—empty beds and shadowy figures pushing empty wheelchairs remain; a lone patient struggles down a dimly lit corridor into darkness, pushing his IV (intravenous) stand with him every step of the way. The video fades abruptly to black, like the plague sucking life out of unwilling individuals far too soon. As for the uninfected others portrayed in scenes with the infected characters, their most striking features are the emotional distance they maintain, and their seemingly unlimited supply of latex gloves.

Because this music video was designed to educate young people about HIV/AIDS and to encourage safer-sex practices, its primary persuasive strategy involves alerting viewers as to what may happen to them if they ignore safer-sex guidelines and, as a result, one day find themselves stricken with full-blown AIDS. Accordingly, it is quite surprising that *all* of the people with AIDS in the music video appear to be significantly older than virtually all members of the target audience, and that *none* of them appear to be just "ordinary people" rather than members of what are stereotypically thought to be the highest-risk groups for contracting HIV and AIDS: gay men, IV drug users, and people in Africa. In short, the lyrics and visual images in the video actually seem to contradict each another. While the lyrics urge recipients of the message to see past all the stereotypes and fear surrounding AIDS and people with AIDS, the visual images serve primarily to reinforce the traditional stereotypes and perceptions of the need for fear.

The music video's exclusive focus on portraying only gay men, IV drug users, and people from Africa as infected suggests that AIDS is of concern, almost exclusively, to members of these groups (which is untrue) (Wright, 1997, pp. 77-79; Yep and Pietri, 1999, p. 199), and the inclusion of latex gloves in every scene mixing infected and uninfected individuals suggests that infected individuals are highly contagious and must definitely be feared (again, untrue). Such a representation makes the people with AIDS in the music video appear to be "twice removed" from the majority of audience members at whom the video is directed. Most of these individuals envision themselves as young and "invincible" and do not picture themselves as part of a demographic group considered to be highly "at risk." Regardless of whether such perceptions are realistic, it is noteworthy that the video makes little attempt to challenge inaccurate and outdated ways of thinking about AIDS and people with AIDS. The question thus arises: Why have the creators of this video chosen to represent AIDS in this way?

Many undergraduate focus group participants at the University of Michigan, Ann Arbor, have argued, after viewing this music video, that such a stereotypical representation of AIDS is required in a filmed creation that lasts less than four minutes, to concisely and effectively tell a story, but that such shorthand stereotypical conventions would be far less common in narrative works of longer duration (Hart, 1997, p. 1). But is this actually the case? The goal of the present study is to analyze the representation of AIDS in narrative creations of significantly longer length. Specifically, this study analyzes American movies released during the first two decades of the AIDS pandemic and theorizes about the likely social ramifications of their various representations of AIDS and people with AIDS.

AIDS, SOCIAL CONSTRUCTION,
AND MEDIA REPRESENTATION

AIDS entered the American consciousness in 1981, during an era of increasing complacency within the medical community regarding infectious diseases (Morse, 1992, p. 23). Just when many doctors believed that infectious diseases would soon be a thing of the past, a few in New York, Los Angeles, and San Francisco began diagnosing a variety of rare opportunistic diseases—including Kaposi's sarcoma (KS) and *Pneumocystis carinii* pneumonia (PCP)—in otherwise healthy gay male patients. At the time, the KS/PCP condition was referred to by physicians as GRID, which stood for "gay-related immune deficiency"; throughout American society, it was more typically referred to as "gay cancer" and the "gay plague." The term *AIDS*, or "acquired immunodeficiency syndrome," was adopted by the Centers for Disease Control (CDC) in 1982, in part to reflect the reality that the disease had appeared in individuals other than gay men, such as hemophiliacs, blood-transfusion recipients, users of intravenous drugs, Haitians who had emigrated to the United States, and newborn babies. The next year, researchers successfully isolated the virus that ravages human immune systems and eventually labeled it HIV, which stands for "human immunodeficiency virus." HIV is one of a relatively small group of viruses known as retroviruses, which attack an infected individual's immune system and render the individual defenseless against a variety of opportunistic diseases (Elwood, 1999, p. vii). It is transmitted primarily through intimate sexual activity, exposure to contaminated blood, and perinatally from mother to child, with the most likely consequence of HIV infection ultimately being death.

Over the past two decades, the HIV/AIDS pandemic has affected all kinds of Americans, including members of sexual minority communities and diverse cultural groups; females and males; children, adolescents, and adults; hemophiliacs; injection drug users and their partners; and heterosexuals, among others (Yep and Pietri, 1999, p. 199). It has become the most common cause of death for American men between the ages of twenty-five and forty-four and a leading cause of death for American women in the same age group (Elwood, 1999, p. vii; *Out Post*, 1998, p. 11). Nevertheless, the process by which AIDS became a pandemic of public proportions has been far from value free (Cook and Colby, 1992, p. 84); each stage of research and treatment has been accompanied by ideological battles over the meaning and social significance of HIV/AIDS (Piontek, 1992, p. 142). To a significant degree, that is because use of the medical term *GRID* served to define AIDS as a gay male disease from the earliest days of the pandemic, even though both heterosexual and homosexual men and women were infected early on (Perrow and Guillen, 1990, p. 3). Although inaccurate, this initial perception of the reality of the AIDS pandemic has proven difficult to overcome, despite the efforts of all sorts of individuals in American society to alter this perceived "reality."

During the 1990s, the demographics of Americans being diag-nosed with AIDS in American society significantly changed: re-ported cases of AIDS resulting from heterosexual transmission of HIV increased steadily, with heterosexual women, heterosexual African-American men, and heterosexual adolescents becoming sizable high-risk groups for HIV transmission and AIDS (Wright, 1997, pp. 77-79). However, many Americans still continue to clas-sify AIDS in their minds as a disease of "the other"—whether that "other" is an intravenous drug user, someone with a "deviant" sexu-al orientation, or someone living on another continent (Netzhammer and Shamp, 1994, p. 98)—thus providing them with a sense of immunity from the pandemic and frequently leading them to avoid preventive behaviors. The social construction of AIDS in American society is largely responsible for this unfortunate state of affairs.

The social-construction perspective maintains that contemporary historical reality does not exist as a truth waiting to be discovered; instead, it is created by a range of social actors in the same society who compete with one another over the appropriate construction of contem-porary historical conditions (Fee and Fox, 1992, p. 9). As a result, the ways in which these social actors communicatively delineate any spe-cific social issue have profound implications for the way a society regards that issue—how other people think about the issue itself, the people associated with that issue, and the appropriate actions (if any) they should take personally with regard to that issue (Elwood, 1999, p. 6). In other words, as Michel Foucault has posited in his various writings, human discourse and social power are inherently intertwined such that discourse ultimately determines the historical conditions experienced by various members of the same society.

As behavioral scientist William Elwood has noted in his summary of Foucault's theorizing, human communication processes among prominent social actors ultimately determine social practices and historical conditions, for they determine what constitutes "truth" and appropriate social actions in any society and promote ways that the self must be molded in response to such dictates (1999, p. 6). This suggests that social actors possessing the greatest degree of social power retain pervasive terminological power to define and influence social issues and conditions. It also suggests that social constructions do not necessarily correspond to reality in any objective sense, even though they continually influence the way individuals perceive the real world and their requisite reactions to it (Rushing, 1995, p. 136). There are real conditions in the world and then there are constructions of those conditions that are presented to us, and that we present to ourselves and others. Social constructions serve to convey a sense of certainty in an uncertain world, and individuals tend to respond to them regardless of their inherent validity (Ibid.).

With regard to AIDS, specifically, communicative interaction among social actors has resulted in the social construction of the pandemic, which in turn has determined the reactions of individuals and American society as a whole toward HIV/AIDS and those already infected. According to the social-construction perspective, individuals respond to AIDS in terms of its social definition—which derives from social and cultural conditions in addition to biological conditions— regardless of the scientific validity of that definition (Rushing, 1995, p. 163). Throughout the history of the pandemic, therefore, the ways in which AIDS and those who have been infected and affected by it have been communicatively constructed have affected transmission and prevention, medical treatment and outcomes, tolerance and compassion (Roth and Fuller, 1998, p. 2). Americans have used these social constructions, however inadequate they may be, to make sense of the pandemic and to guide their personal responses to it. Stemming from Althusserian notions of ideology, gender studies scholar Cindy Patton has referred to this process as the "invention" of AIDS (1990, p. 77). By this, she means that the shared social understanding of the pandemic results from the totality of stories that Americans tell themselves about HIV/AIDS, with stories disseminated by more powerful and authoritative sources most fully shaping that understanding. Similarly, cultural critic Douglas Crimp has concluded that AIDS, as a social and medical phenomenon, can only be fully comprehended through an understanding of the practices and strategies that conceptualize and represent HIV/AIDS (1987, p. 3). For example, the decision to refer to infected individuals as either AIDS victims, AIDS sufferers, AIDS patients, or people with AIDS can have profound social implications.

Whether it occurs between small groups of people or millions, communication of social constructions serves as a primary means by which individuals influence others in their social world about various issues. As such, media representations of social phenomena contribute significantly to widely shared social perceptions. "In a society that spans a continent, in a cosmopolitan culture which spans much of the globe," explains media scholar Larry Gross, "the mass media provide the broadest common background of assumptions about what things are, how they work (or should work), and why" (1994, p. 143). Gross elaborates on this point by noting that mainstream media offerings are typically presented to audience members as "transparent mediators of reality" in the social world, and that even the most sophisticated of media users can identify components of their "knowledge" of the real world that derive either wholly or significantly from media representations, fictional or otherwise (Ibid., p. 144).

Because media representations use culturally shared codes and conventions to communicate social information, they simultaneously enable and restrict what individuals can say about any aspect of "reality" in a given society at a given time (Dyer, 1993, p. 2). Although recent research efforts in the cultural-studies tradition have revealed that the meanings delivered by media representations are not determined entirely by the mediated texts or their producers, the use of such culturally shared codes and conventions helps to delimit the range of interpretations that can effectively be achieved. In other words, the "openness" of interpretation inherent in models of message encoding and decoding actually has practical limits, making it unlikely that the majority of receivers will be able to interpret most mediated texts significantly differently from the way they are intended by their senders (Hart, 1999, p. 210).

The treatment of AIDS in news accounts, documentaries, television programs, movies, and other mass media offerings over the past two decades has undeniably shaped the way the American public thinks about and responds, socially and politically, to the pandemic. Media representations have shaped the social processes and semantics under-lying all aspects of the pandemic, including conceptions of risk, vul-nerability, drug use, and sexuality; accordingly, these representations have had a direct bearing on the already complex relationships within and between various social groups (Estrada and Quintero, 1999, p. 133). Once these mediated social constructions become part of the American social agenda, they become the commonly accepted ways to discuss HIV and AIDS, and they influence whether individuals per-ceive themselves to be at risk for contracting or transmitting HIV/ AIDS and how they respond to others with and without HIV/AIDS (Elwood, 1999, p. 416). Media representations of AIDS provide ideo-logical guidance to American audience members; as such, the codes, conventions, symbols, and visuals they offer contribute significantly to the social construction of the pandemic and to the social ramifications of that construction. For better or worse, representational practices mold a society's cultural relationship to the AIDS pandemic, both directly and indirectly influencing the pandemic's present and future realities (Erni, 1994, p. 114).

DEFINING AND ANALYZING THE AIDS MOVIE

To date, systematic studies of media representations of AIDS have restricted themselves primarily to print media (especially newspapers and newsmagazines), television news, and prime-time television shows (Cook and Colby, 1992, p. 86; Netzhammer and Shamp, 1994, p. 92). The present study extends prior research by focusing on represen-tations of AIDS in American movies, which offer unique opportunities for the presentation of more personalized, vivid, and memorable mes-sages about AIDS and people with AIDS (Cook and Colby, 1992, p. 88). It is intended to provide the most comprehensive study of the cultural phenomenon of movies about AIDS that has yet been at-tempted. The guiding research question of this study is, In what ways do movies about HIV/AIDS influence American ideology and contribute to the ongoing social construction and reconstruction of the pandemic?

In much the same way that film scholars refer to groups of movies as being examples of "prison movies" (movies focused around the theme of civil imprisonment, which either are set primarily within prison walls or explore the anguish and suffering resulting from incarceration) or "road movies" (movies focused around the theme of exploration on the road, which lead central characters to intriguing locations and explore the social, political, and cultural realities encountered during their journeys), I use the term *AIDS movie* in this study to refer to any fictional or fictionalized narrative movie which features at least one character who either (1) has been infected with HIV, (2) has developed full-blown AIDS, and/or (3) is grieving the recent death of a loved one from AIDS and which also explores the process of such characters confronting realities associated with transmitting, living with, and/or dying from HIV or AIDS as a significant component of its narrative. Consistent with previous research on the representation of AIDS in American movies, therefore, the term *AIDS* is being used in this study "to refer both to the condition of infection with the human [immunodeficiency] virus (HIV/HIV infection) and to the condition of anyone experiencing the multiple disease pattern referred to as acquired immune [deficiency] syndrome (AIDS)" (Pilipp and Shull, 1993, p. 19).

In this study, movies that are "based on a true story"—such as *The Ryan White Story* (1989), *Citizen Cohn* (1992), and *Gia* (1998)—qualify for inclusion as AIDS movies because they are fictionalized accounts and typically contain disclaimers to alert viewers of their fictionalized nature. For example, the disclaimer at the end of *Gia* explains that the film is a dramatization of actual events in which some of the characters and events have been fictionalized to heighten the drama. Similar disclaimers alert viewers to the presence of characters, dialogue, and events that are composites or entirely fictional creations. In contrast, movies that introduce only supporting characters with HIV or AIDS, and do so in a way that is incidental to the plot; movies that are constructed to serve as metaphors for HIV/AIDS infection rather than explicit representations of HIV/AIDS infection; and movies that are documentaries about HIV or AIDS do not qualify as narrative AIDS movies in this study, although such offerings will be discussed in the concluding chapter as examples of alternative representational approaches. In addition, to ensure that sound theory building can be attempted in the tradition of American cultural studies, only movies produced in the United States qualify for inclusion in this study. Finally, to ensure that feature-length movies remain the focus of this project, as intended, this study established an a priori (and somewhat arbitrary) forty-five-minute minimum length requirement for movies to qualify for inclusion. Hundreds of short films about AIDS ranging in length from thirty seconds to several minutes have been produced in the United States over the past two decades and are quite worthy of research attention, but they provide the foundation for another research project (or, indeed, several) entirely, as they have been far less central to the social construction of AIDS in American society than the offerings analyzed here.

Some of the most significant ramifications of recent advancements in media technology include the exponential increase in the sheer volume of images that are transmitted to and playable in the average American household, as well as the ever-expanding circulation and recirculation of signs that form the fabric of American cultural life (Collins, 1993, p. 246). Because the traditional distinctions that existed between theatrical releases and made-for-television movies have largely been eradicated with the widespread availability of cable television, videocassette recorders (VCRs), and prerecorded videocassette/DVD (digital versatile disc) retail and rental outlets in recent years—and because concerns regarding the social effects of media representations revolve primarily around cumulative exposure to related representations more so than exposure to individual, isolated ones—this study devotes equivalent attention to theatrical releases (both mainstream and independent), made-for-cable movies, and made-for-television movies.

The present study takes a cultural-studies approach to analyzing the representation of AIDS in American movies produced during the first two decades of the AIDS pandemic and to theorizing about the likely social ramifications of those representations. Accordingly, it involves an interdisciplinary approach to the study of the production and circulation of meanings pertaining to AIDS in American culture, ultimately investigating and theorizing about the relations between culture and society that inherently involve issues of status and power (Byars,

1991, p. 39). This study proceeds from a definition of culture that refers to the historically distinct values and viewpoints that define a society at a specific period in time and the social processes used to widely disseminate those values and viewpoints (Ibid., p. 40). Consistent with related research endeavors in the cultural-studies tradition, it insists on the centrality of social constructionism in molding public perceptions of, and reactions to, this chronic disease, maintaining that public responses to AIDS and people with AIDS are determined partially, yet significantly, by the internal logic and workings of the mass media (Fee and Fox, 1992, p. 14).

More specifically, this study combines the empirical advantages of social-scientific content analysis with the theoretical flexibility of humanistic textual analysis and criticism, within a cultural-studies framework. The majority of the study involves extensive analysis of the manifest contents of AIDS movies released during the 1980s and 1990s. Because no comprehensive list of such movies appears to exist, a three-month period was devoted to compiling one using indexes and descriptions in numerous film and video guides, scholarly and popular writings about media portrayals of HIV and AIDS, and various Internet sites. These efforts produced a list of forty movies (see Appendix A) meeting the criteria in the aforementioned definition of an AIDS movie. Although the researcher's initial goal was to analyze all of these movies, a subsequent six-month search revealed that eight of these titles were unavailable for analysis, either for viewing, rental, or purchase. Accordingly, the analysis conducted in this study is based on the thirty-two AIDS movies (see Appendix B) that were available; textual materials pertaining to the remaining eight movies suggest that their overall contents are not qualitatively different from the contents of the movies analyzed here.

The thirty-two analyzed movies were examined with regard to the demographic characteristics (gender, sexual orientation, age category, race/ethnicity) and infection status (HIV/AIDS) of characters identified to be infected with HIV or AIDS, explanations of how such characters contracted HIV/AIDS, evidence of victim blaming, and the ultimate status of each character identified to be infected with HIV/AIDS at movie's end. The findings are presented in the following four chapters, which are centered around the theme of "otherness and the AIDS movie." Chapter 2 discusses the cinematic tradition of otherness and its

relation to the AIDS movie. Chapter 3 examines the cultural phenomenon of "innocent victims" and the politics of victim blaming in the
AIDS movie. Chapter 4 explores the persistent representation of gay
men as "the other" in the AIDS movie. Chapter 5 addresses the representation of the city (versus the country) in the AIDS movie as yet
another noteworthy form of otherness influencing the ongoing social
construction and reconstruction of the AIDS pandemic in American
society. Additional specifics about the research methods employed in
this study are presented in these chapters.

The concluding chapter of this project, titled "Other Ways of Representing AIDS," explores alternative approaches to representing AIDS
in American movies. It begins with an exploration of the form and
function of AIDS characters in "non-AIDS movies," fictional offerings
that include at least one character with HIV/AIDS yet do so in ways
that are incidental to their narratives. In other words, these movies
could delete all references to HIV/AIDS and achieve similar narrative
ends using different narrative means without significantly altering their
plots. From there, the chapter proceeds to examine AIDS metaphor
movies, fictional offerings that do not explicitly represent HIV/AIDS
yet are encoded to serve as metaphors for HIV/AIDS infection. Next, it
explores the self-representation of people with AIDS in AIDS documentaries. Each of these unique kinds of movies is analyzed with
regard to its comparative strengths and shortcomings in the quest to
accurately represent AIDS and people with AIDS in American society.
Finally, the chapter concludes with an update on the current status of
HIV/AIDS transmission in the United States and the resulting need to
continue representing AIDS during the third decade of the AIDS pandemic and (likely) beyond.

SIGNIFICANCE OF THE STUDY

Mass-mediated texts are widely regarded as central sites for the
struggle over social meaning in industrialized societies (Byars, 1991,
p. 6). With respect to the United States, specifically, there is no denying that the mass media exert significant social power in American
society. A noteworthy dimension of this power is the ability to as-
semble and disseminate social constructions that frequently become
the perceived "reality" of audience members. Accordingly, as modern

studies scholar Thomas Piontek has noted, any solid analysis of the media representation of AIDS must confront the social construction of the pandemic and the resulting meanings ascribed to it, since no representation is ever free of social construction (1992, pp. 128, 144).

To date, movies about AIDS largely have been overlooked as the subject of research investigation, even though preliminary findings in the field of media studies suggest that viewers' parasocial interaction with characters in entertainment offerings provides such offerings with special opportunities to influence people's perceptions of AIDS and those who are infected and affected by the pandemic (Cathcart, 1986, p. 207; Netzhammer and Shamp, 1994, p. 91). Also, preliminary experimental findings in the field of social psychology suggest that fictional portrayals can be more influential in the formation of beliefs about members of social groups that are relatively unfamiliar to audience members than nonfictional portrayals (Slater, 1990, p. 343). Over the past two decades, AIDS movies have taken viewers—many of whom may not yet personally know anyone with HIV/AIDS—to "otherwise inaccessible backstages of individual motivation, organizational performance, and subcultural life" (Gross, 1994, p. 144). Furthermore, it has been acknowledged that media representations can be especially powerful in cultivating images of groups and phenomena about which viewers have little firsthand knowledge, especially when such representations are not readily contradicted by other culturally pervasive beliefs and ideologies (Ibid.).

Movies about AIDS are themselves "constructions" rather than "reflections" of conditions in American society. They disseminate information about the kinds of people who are infected (and at risk of infection) with HIV/AIDS, where these people come from, how they live, what they think and feel, and how others respond to their needs (Watney, 1996, p. 123). In the process, they open up, encourage, and attempt to close down certain audience member decodings in identifiable ways, through their narrative contents, formal elements, codes and conventions, and representations of social reality (Byars, 1991, p. 64). This study identifies such ways and their likely social ramifications, all the while acknowledging that representation is a form of social action involving the production of meanings that ultimately have real effects.

Chapter 2

The Cinematic Tradition of Otherness Meets AIDS

Otherness has been central to the cinematic tradition since the early days of motion pictures. Westerns, for example, which are typically traced back to Edwin S. Porter's 1903 movie *The Great Train Robbery*, are based entirely around the concept of otherness—hero versus villain, civilization versus savagery, individualism versus democracy, strength versus weakness, garden versus desert. A core appeal of screwball comedies, which originated in the mid-1930s, as well as numerous musicals, is the need to reconcile the seemingly irreconcilable otherness of their romantic leads, who typically come from very different class backgrounds. A major draw of films noir, which became quite popular in the 1940s and 1950s, is the concealed otherness of one or more central characters, who ultimately reveal their darker sides as the narratives progress, to the detriment of the protagonists. One form of otherness in slasher movies, which peaked in popularity during the 1970s and 1980s, serves to determine who will live and who must die—those who commit the sin of premarital fornication must pay the price for their "illicit" and "deviant" ways.

Otherness has also been associated with AIDS from the earliest days of the pandemic—AIDS populations have been distinguished from the general population, risk groups from groups not at risk, innocent victims from guilty ones, contaminated blood from pure blood (Gamson, 1989, pp. 359-360). When the first AIDS movies—the made-for-television movie *An Early Frost* about a young gay lawyer with AIDS who comes out to his family, and the independent theatrical movie *Buddies* about a politically vocal gay AIDS patient and his volunteer male counselor and "buddy"—were released in 1985, they certainly did not emerge from a creative moviemaking vacuum. As such, it is perhaps unsurprising that the representation of otherness in those AIDS movies, and many others since, is similar in identifiable ways to the representation of otherness in other kinds of movies. The representation of otherness in AIDS movies resembles the representation of otherness in Westerns, for example, by incorporating binary oppositions (e.g., good/evil) and taking them to new extremes (innocence/guilt, contamination/purity, implicated/immune, us/them). In addition, the representation of otherness in AIDS movies resembles the representation of otherness in slasher movies by incorporating the trope of punishment for illicit sex and linking it to certain types of "morally deviant" others.

What is likely already clear from this brief discussion is that the concept of otherness is defined and applied somewhat differently in various contexts and by various theorists. With regard to the process of media representation, in general, however, the term *otherness* typically refers to the status of certain kinds of individuals being constructed as marginal to, or deviant from, members of the social mainstream in noteworthy ways, as well as certain social phenomena being constructed as marginal to, or deviant from, the social mainstream status quo. As a result, media representations of otherness regularly engage feelings, for example, fears and anxieties, about "the other" in relation to the self and/or in relation to mainstream social norms (Hall, 1997, p. 226). In this regard, the representation of otherness in AIDS movies is most similar to the representation of otherness in two particular kinds of movies: science fiction movies and melodramas.

Parallels between the representation of otherness in these two kinds of movies and the representation of otherness in AIDS movies is the focus of the present chapter. Because it is acknowledged that many readers of this work may have viewed only a handful of AIDS movies to date, the primary goal of the discussion that follows is to begin to define more fully the narrative form of the AIDS movie (with regard to its representational strategies) by comparing and contrasting it with the two narrative forms to which it is most similar regarding the representation of otherness, and with which many readers are likely more familiar. To most efficiently facilitate this discussion, well-known movies that are widely regarded as being representative of the offerings in their respective genres serve to provide the primary examples of the representational approaches under examination.

OTHERNESS, SCIENCE FICTION, AND AIDS

The origins of science fiction movies are traced back to the turn-of-the-century films of Georges Melies. Although an agreed-upon definition of the phrase *science fiction* has somewhat eluded researchers and scholars, it is generally accepted that science fiction movies deal with yet-unknown (or, at the very least, not yet fully known) journeys, worlds, and social conditions presented from the standpoint of credible possibility in rational scientific terms (Lopez, 1993, p. 267). Typically, science fiction movies deal with humans' hopes and fears for the fate of civilization and about what lies beyond known boundaries, and they usually emphasize the unusual and/or the unknown (Parish and Pitts, 1977, p. vii). The ultimate threat in such movies is frequently the destruction of life as we know it, as a result of some noteworthy deviation from the main-stream status quo (Shapiro, 1990, p. 111). As such, it is relatively easy to identify the most significant similarities between representations of otherness in science fiction movies and representations of otherness in AIDS movies, which also focus, in their own way, on hopes and fears for the fate of human civilization and a scientifically credible threat to life as we know it.

Although it comes in various forms, otherness is an essential component of science fiction narratives. One common form of otherness represented in science fiction movies materializes through the structured encouragement of viewer comparisons between present-day realities and those provided on screen, with regard to deviations from current mainstream social conditions and norms. Consider the representation of otherness in *THX 1138*, the first science fiction offering from director George Lucas, for example. Released in 1971, *THX 1138* offers a startling vision of the world of tomorrow, one in which dehumanization and mandatory conformity pervade a huge subterranean colony in which everybody and everything is controlled by computers, and residents are forced to ingest powerful sedatives to keep them in their submissive state. It presents a world in which all people look alike, dress alike, act alike, and are identified by numbers rather than names, and in which futuristic robot police roam the land, enforcing the desires of the state. After LUH 3417 (played by Maggie McOmie) sees through all the social rhetoric and realizes the kind of oppressive society in which she is trapped, she discontinues her daily tranquilizers and alters the sedative intake of her male roommate, THX 1138 (played by Robert Duvall), as well. Freed from the chemical ties that bind, they break the law by falling in love and having sex; LUH 3417 becomes pregnant. During the same period, SEN 5241 (Donald Pleasence) enacts a plan to modify the colony's computerized roommate-matching system, desiring to pair himself with THX 1138. Ultimately, all three are turned over to the authorities and found guilty of their offenses. LUH 3417 is sentenced to death; THX 1138 and SEN 5241 bide their time in a prisonlike, seemingly endless white void, plotting their escape. Although both successfully make their way out of the imprisoning whiteness and into the city, it is only THX 1138 who survives pursuit by the robotic police, emerging from a ventilator shaft and greeting the outside world. A brilliant sunset welcomes him as he begins a new life's journey.

Certainly, the otherness represented in *THX 1138* becomes fully comprehensible only after the viewer compares current social realities in American society with those which could one day be experienced if present trends continue unchecked and unabated over the course of the next few centuries. In movies such as this one, the psychological appeal of the otherness encountered results primarily from the recognition that it is the potential end result of the world of our creation and the fact that we created it (Shapiro, 1990, p. 109). A similar sort of appeal can be identified in most AIDS movies, which implies that the unfortunate health realities being experienced by increasing numbers of individuals with every passing year are the human-made end result of more permissive sexual mores, stemming from the days of free love in the 1960s and beyond. The ideological implications contained in both of these kinds of movies, therefore, are discernible only after the viewer identifies the relatively "unseen terrors that lurk beneath the surface normality" of modern American society and contemplates where they ultimately could one day lead (Ibid., p. 105).

A far more straightforward and more readily interpretable incarnation of otherness in science fiction movies is that of "the other," which can range from physical beings (aliens, monsters) that are clearly deviant from members of the social mainstream to social phenomena (such as conditions and diseases that endanger human lives) that deviate significantly from the social mainstream status quo. A classic example of the other is found in the 1956 science fiction movie *Invasion of the Body Snatchers,* in the form of seeds drifting through space that enter Earth's atmosphere, take hold in a farmer's field, and reproduce themselves as exact likenesses of other living beings, threatening the well-being of the entire human race as we know it. In this movie, Dr. Miles Bennell (played by Kevin McCarthy) and his romantic interest, Becky Driscoll (played by Dana Wynter), are among a handful of residents in a quaint Northern California community to notice that their fellow townspeople are inevitably being transformed by the seeds into emotionless, zombielike beings. As the narrative unfolds, Miles and Becky realize that giant seedpods containing look-alikes of their fellow residents—and ultimately of themselves—are growing everywhere around them, taking over the minds and bodies of humans while they sleep and leaving unfeeling duplicates in their place. Confronted with their own pods, Miles and Becky are informed that their new bodies will take them over cell for cell, engulfing their minds and memories, causing them to be reborn into an untroubled world in the process. Note the similarity between the effect of the seedpods on individuals in this science fiction movie and the effect of HIV on individuals in AIDS movies, who similarly are taken over cell by cell until they are reborn (spiritually) into another life.

Additional examples of the threatening other in science fiction movies, among many others, include radioactivity from atomic warfare that is wiping out humanity worldwide in *On the Beach* (1959) and an alien microorganism that falls to Earth and threatens to eradicate all life forms coming into its proximity in *The Andromeda Strain* (1971).

By now, the representational parallels between the other in science fiction movies and the other in AIDS movies should be increasingly apparent because a recurring narrative strategy in science fiction movies—as in AIDS movies—involves the graphic revealing of the physical effects on humans exposed to the other as it wreaks its social havoc, whether by dramatic physical transformations (as in the 1957 science fiction movie *The Amazing Colossal Man*) or the process of dying and death (as in the 1924 science fiction movie *The Last Man on Earth* and the aforementioned *On the Beach*). In other words, the initial other that surfaces within the social world ultimately transforms healthy human beings into alternate versions of themselves, or a second form of the other. With regard to AIDS movies, therefore, the initial form of the other is typically the HIV virus, and the graphic revealing of the physical effects on humans exposed to the virus—especially as it progresses to full-blown AIDS and beyond—transforms formerly healthy human beings into living, breathing, compromised variations of themselves, or "the other" version of their former selves.

Perhaps the most startling example of this process occurs in the 1993 AIDS movie *Philadelphia*, which stars Tom Hanks as Andrew Beckett, an HIV-infected lawyer who becomes politicized after encountering homophobia and AIDS discrimination in the workplace. When the viewer first glimpses Beckett, he is a remarkably vibrant and healthy-looking man; little does the viewer know that the other, in the form of HIV, has already invaded his body. Soon, however, the first sign that Beckett's transformation into a compromised version of himself has begun appears on his forehead: a KS lesion. As the narrative proceeds, and the other becomes increasingly powerful within Beckett's system, the character's body physically deteriorates and appears as though it has aged the equivalent of several decades in only a few months, with his dark brown hair becoming as white as an elderly man's, and his physique becoming increasingly frail. On his hospital deathbed, Beckett is but a shadow of his former self—a second form of the other—and he is so weak that he can barely move or speak.

Returning to the discussion of parallels between otherness in science fiction movies and AIDS movies, as demonstrated through the example of *Invasion of the Body Snatchers*, it is noteworthy that Dr. Miles Bennell flees the location of his own seedpod in search of help before that narrative concludes, taking Becky Driscoll with him. After Becky reluctantly falls asleep and becomes one of "them," Miles is left to try to save the rest of the world on his own.

According to the logic of science fiction movies, however, he is among the limited number of individuals in society who retain the greatest potential ability to do so. It is certainly no coincidence that the narrative of this movie revolves around the discoveries of a medical doctor, thereby tapping into the aura of scientific credibility; a noteworthy narrative pattern in science fiction movies involves attempts by doctors and scientists to save individuals threatened by the other, to make a valiant effort at rescuing a person or a world on the brink of disaster (Shapiro, 1990, p. 106). The assumption in science fiction movies is that science will save humanity if anything can, yet it is not atypical for movies of this kind to leave viewers wondering if the individuals or communities presented in the movie will actually survive in the future (Sobchack, 1995, p. 111).

Within AIDS movies, medical science is similarly presented as making committed attempts at finding a cure and saving individuals threatened by the other. The 1985 AIDS movie *An Early Frost*, for example, vividly reveals the lack of knowledge about the disease, experienced by medical professionals in gripping scenes during which emergency personnel are terrified to transport a person with AIDS (played by Aidan Quinn), or when doctors sincerely do not know how to treat him. The 1991 AIDS movie *Jerker*, a drama in which two San Francisco gay men engage in anonymous phone sex on a regular basis during the early years of the AIDS pandemic—when phone sex was considered to be the only truly safe sex—demonstrates how quickly the other can claim the life of the human being it inhabits, despite ongoing efforts by medical science to eradicate it, even when that individual shows few outward signs of illness. In that movie, Bert (played by Tom Wagner) dies quite suddenly, within days after it becomes obvious that he is infected with HIV/ AIDS, and in spite of the best efforts by doctors to prolong the lives of individuals like him. The 1993 AIDS movie *And the Band Played On*, based on Randy Shilts's (1987) controversial book about the AIDS pandemic, details the extensive efforts made by doctors in the United States and France to isolate and hopefully eradicate the other, the seemingly insurmountable virus that has baffled medical science for years. The 1997 AIDS movie *In the Gloaming* reveals the ultimate outcome when medical science has failed in its attempts to rescue an individual on the brink of a health disaster, as a grown son (played by Robert Sean Leonard) returns home to his family to make peace and die. Similar to science fiction movies, these AIDS movies and many others offer the hope that science will ultimately save humanity, yet as a result of past and relatively unchanged present realities associated with the AIDS pandemic, they leave viewers suspecting that the individuals presented will be unable to survive for long.

Although much was known by medical scientists about the interaction of viruses with the human immune system in the early 1980s, the otherness of HIV emerged as powerfully distinct: a virus that causes human disease by depleting the cells responsible for immunity from disease was unprecedented (Morse, 1992, p. 24). In journalistic and biomedical discourses from the earliest days of the AIDS pandemic to the present, therefore, the otherness of HIV has been described variously as "a brilliant genetic design that facilitates undetectable infection"; "the invading battalion, turning the body into a war zone"; a powerful force with the formidable "ability to claim territories and remain there to reproduce its own kind"; and of an origin that is "unmistakably foreign and alien" (Erni, 1994, p. 41). Similarly, descriptions of HIV in the popular media have commonly adopted the language of science fiction to infuse themselves with immediate audience appeal. Accordingly, it seems quite logical that AIDS movies, from their inception, would come to resemble science fiction movies in identifiable ways. At the same time, representations of otherness in AIDS movies also differ from representations of otherness in science fiction movies in significant ways.

Movies featuring encounters with the other are the most common type of science fiction offering; ideologically, the cumulative message these movies send is that otherness is threatening to human life and to social mores (Hayward, 1996, p. 305). Because the other in such movies is generally a creation of the science fiction imagination that comes from outer space, however, few people complain about the appropriateness or inappropriateness of its representation in American science fiction offerings. As film scholar Richard Maltby has summarized this state of affairs, "In space, no one can hear you scream about misrepresentation" (1995, p. 132). It is not surprising, therefore, that the other in science fiction movies is incorporated primarily to produce anxiety in viewers over the circumstances characters may potentially encounter, and that it is consistently presented in such a way as to *never* evoke viewer sympathy (Sobchack, 1997, pp. 32, 39). The ideological and social implications of such representational approaches, however, change dramatically when the science fiction hallmark of the other appears in similar fashion in AIDS movies, and this other (in the form of the HIV virus) systematically transforms a living, breathing, healthy human being into a second form of the other, known as a person with AIDS.

The regular representation of HIV as the other in AIDS movies, which gradually yet inadvertently transforms human beings simultaneously into alternate versions of both the other and themselves, introduces the need, unlike in works of science fiction, for viewers potentially to experience significant levels of viewer sympathy in response to the on-screen other. In such movies, the fear surrounding infection with HIV/AIDS is represented as both the fear of the other and, ultimately, of the self, with the self simultaneously being a second form of the other (which is undeserving of viewer sympathy) as well as an endangered human being (who therefore is much deserving of viewer sympathy). The question thus arises: Under what conditions do viewers of AIDS movies resist experiencing sympathy for characters with HIV/AIDS because they view such characters primarily as the other, and under what conditions do viewers of AIDS movies more readily and more willingly experience sympathy for characters with HIV/AIDS because they view such characters primarily as human beings deserving of such a response? The answer to this question lies in the exploration of the relatively common, binary oppositional construction of "innocent victims" and "guilty villains" in AIDS movies, which is discussed at length in Chapter 3.

OTHERNESS, MELODRAMA, AND AIDS

The origins of melodramas lie not in the cinema but, rather, have been deeply rooted in Western culture since the eighteenth century, in the theater and in prose fiction (Landy, 1991, p. 15). When silent cinema appeared, melodrama served as an ideal form of content because of its ability to work on a purely emotional level, rooting its drama in visual expression and conveying its emotion effectively through various elements of mise-en-scène (Belton, 1994, p. 117). D. W. Griffith emerged as the master of the silent melodrama, establishing its style, tone, and substance in movies, including *Broken Blossoms* (1919) and *Way Down East* (1920) (Schatz, 1991, p. 149). The addition of sound in the late 1920s transformed the melodrama from the format by which the majority of movies were made into a distinct genre among many (Belton, 1994, p. 132). Hollywood filmmakers began increasingly to test the range and emotional power of melodramatic narratives, and their affective appeal to audience members became undeniable (Schatz, 1991, p. 149). The narrative emphases in melodramas involve interrelated families of characters, repressive small-town milieus, and preoccupation with Americans' sociosexual mores (Ibid., p. 151). Although melodramas traditionally have featured women as their protagonists, the genre continued to evolve in recent decades with movies such as *Kramer vs. Kramer* (1979) and *Ordinary People* (1980) in which men (often fathers), rather than women, began serving as the main protagonists in melodramatic works (Maltby, 1995, p. 223; Britton, 1986, p. 24). Overall, melodramas are associated in contemporary critical discourse with stories of family trauma, pathos, and heightened emotionalism (Maltby, 1995, p. 133).

Otherness in melodramas typically manifests itself in the form of a character who deviates in a readily identifiable way from surrounding others in the patriarchal social order. In the 1937 melodrama *Stella Dallas,* for example, this character is Stella herself (played by Barbara Stanwyck), an ambitious, lower-class woman who marries a wealthy businessman after convincing him that she wants him to provide her education into upper-class society. Shortly after the birth of the couple's only child, a daughter named Laurel (whom Stella calls "Lolly"), it becomes clear that Stella is not sincere in her quest to become socially refined; she begins to reject the teachings of her husband Stephen (played by John Boles), feeling constrained by his recommendations about how she should dress and behave. Eventually, Stephen becomes disillusioned with his wife, and he leaves both mother and daughter behind in their Massachusetts home when he accepts a job in New York City. It is there, when his daughter is thirteen years old, that Stephen runs into his old flame, Helen Morrison. Now widowed, Mrs. Morrison and her three sons take to the man, and the couple's romance blossoms unhindered. Although Stephen retains his love of his daughter, his disillusionment with the girl's unrefined mother and with Stella's inappropriate suitor, the equally unrefined Ed Munn, continues to grow.

Over the course of the narrative, despite the fact that Stella loves her daughter immensely and would do anything for her, it becomes evident that Stella's unrefined nature is a detriment to the teen. An early example of this occurs on the day of Laurel's birthday party, when all of the invited guests make excuses rather than actually attend. This reoccurs more devastatingly a few years later when Stella takes her daughter on vacation at an elegant countryside resort. Although Stella is sick and bedridden for the first few days of their trip, she certainly makes her presence known when she ventures out of her room in a quest to meet the mother of the young man with whom Laurel is becoming romantically involved. Suffice it to say Stella definitely turns heads with her appearance, yet for all of the wrong reasons. In contrast to her daughter's conservative fashions, Stella wanders about in an outlandish costume, featuring loud patterns, ruffles, a fur wrap, a giant bow in her hair, and a veil covering her face. One of her teenage observers accurately declares that Stella looks like "a Christmas tree," and this is the first time the viewer detects Laurel's embarrassment at her mother's behavior.

At Laurel's insistence, she and Stella depart for home immediately. Late that night, on the train, both Laurel and Stella hear a group of young girls laughing and joking about Stella's outrageous behavior. It is at that moment that Stella launches a plan to divorce Stephen and allow him to marry Mrs. Morrison, so that Laurel can be raised in more proper surroundings, as part of a more traditional family structure. Stella visits her husband's true love to run the idea past her. Mrs. Morrison is touched by the extent of the unselfish sacrifice Stella is willing to make for her daughter.

After arriving for a visit with Stephen and his new bride, Laurel remains committed to the idea of remaining with her mother. Although she thanks them for inviting her to move in, Laurel declares that her home will always be with Stella. That said, Laurel catches a train back to Stella's apartment, and the couple sends Stella a telegram to inform her about the latest developments. In one of the most selfless acts ever seen in movies, Stella forces herself to say hurtful things to Laurel, and she behaves in ways that are quite unappealing: smoking cigarettes, listening to jazz music, and flipping through a common woman's magazine, Stella informs her daughter that she has always wanted to be more in life than simply a mother, and that she has wasted the best years of her life in that role. Laurel is revolted by her mother's actions and devastated by her words; the final straw comes when Stella informs her that she is planning to marry Ed Munn, whom Stella had promised never to become involved with again.

The movie ends with the marriage of Laurel to her young suitor, with Stella viewing the ceremony clearly through the outside window before walking off into the night, smiling but alone. Why does it inevitably have to end this way? Because the most common theme in melodramas is that of the "sacrificial other," the character who deviates in an identifiable way from surrounding others and who restores the patriarchal social order at tremendous personal expense. In this instance, Stella Dallas serves as rebel to the patriarchal social order throughout the film, an individual who, despite her best efforts, never quite fits in. She is a woman of excess in her personal style, and, ultimately, her excessive nature begins to negatively affect the perceived life chances of the daughter she loves so dearly. By making her ultimate self-sacrifice, Stella enables Laurel to live in a home with her father, and as part of a solid family unit. She also enables her daughter to resume her proper place in society, as Laurel is given away at the wedding by Stephen, and the patriarchal order is firmly reestablished.

Because of Stella's isolation at movie's end, it is somewhat difficult to consider this a "happy ending." Yet, within the typical melodrama, it is precisely that. Otherness in melodramas is constructed intentionally to keep the worlds of "normalcy" and of "deviance" iconographically and narratively distinct (Dyer, 1993, p. 102). The primary drive of melodramas is to identify moral polarities of good and evil and, ultimately, to reinforce what is socially good while simultaneously eliminating what is socially evil during an entertaining "drama of morality," in which social "truths," ideologies, and ethics are articulated (Byars, 1991, pp. 11, 18). This means that melodramas strive intentionally to eradicate social otherness within the movie world, for better or for worse.

The 1939 movie *Dark Victory* provides a second example of the way that melodramas present—then seek to contain—otherness in a patriarchal social world. In this melodrama, Bette Davis plays Judith Traherne, a spoiled, fun-loving socialite who discovers that she is dying of a brain tumor. Unlike Stella Dallas, Judith Traherne fits comfortably in the world of upper-class society. Judith's otherness stems instead from the reality that she is a fiery, independent, undomesticated woman who does not seem to need a man (Klaprat, 1985, p. 363). Early in the movie, it becomes clear that although Judith enjoys appealing to and partying with men, she does not want or need one to call her own. After undergoing what she believes to have been a successful operation on her brain, however, she finds herself quite appreciative and begins to fall in love with her surgeon, Dr. Frederick Steele (played by George Brent). The romance does not last long; Judith soon learns that both Frederick and her closest friend, Ann (played by Geraldine Fitzgerald), have been withholding the information that Judith has less than one year left to live, and she distances herself from both of them. With the days of her life slowly drawing to a close, Judith returns to her typical lifestyle in the fast lane.

Unable to stand the waiting, day and night, until her ultimate demise, Judith contemplates suicide. According to the logic of melodramas, however, committing suicide would only increase Judith's otherness—enhancing her status as a fiery, independent, undomesticated women who does not need a man—rather than enable her to make a supreme sacrifice that will restore the patriarchal social order within the story world. As such, it is not entirely surprising to the viewer when Judith begs Frederick's forgiveness, admitting to him that she is afraid and needs his strength. As Judith clutches him and begins to cry, Frederick proposes marriage. Judith's acceptance of his proposal suggests that she is giving up her "deviant" ways and finally adhering to the social expectation of the times—that a woman requires the support, protection, and comfort of a good man.

The movie concludes in Vermont on a beautiful spring day, where Frederick, Judith, and their two dogs have established a home together. Ann is visiting the couple, and she is with Judith when Judith's eyesight begins to fail, indicating that the end is near. Ann breaks down immediately, and Judith comforts her. Although Judith was expected to leave town that afternoon with Frederick to attend a professional gathering, she now asks her husband to travel without her. Not wanting Frederick to perceive that anything is amiss, she feels her way up the staircase using the railing as a guide, and she packs his suitcase by feeling her way around the room. After asking if she has been a good wife, she embraces Frederick on the front lawn and bids him farewell. It becomes clear that, even in her final moments, Judith remains an independent woman who never really needed a man to protect and comfort her, despite the outward appearances of the couple's relationship. Ann cries after Frederick departs; Judith comforts her friend again and says good-bye, emphasizing the importance of her dying alone. Feeling her way back into the house, she says good-bye to her dogs, informs the maid that she does not wish to be disturbed, and guides her way into her bed upstairs. There, she lies down and faces the end of her life on her own, and on her own terms. Judith sacrifices her own emotional needs to minimize the emotionality of her death on her closest loved ones; simultaneously, the patriarchal social order is restored through the eradication of a "deviant" woman who threatens it by remaining independent of any man.

Dark Victory is one of a subgroup of melodramas that focuses on an individual confronting a fatal disease; other representative examples include *Jezebel* (1938) and *Imitation of Life* (1959). In *Jezebel,* a young woman's persistent rejection of her expected, subservient role in relation to men costs her the opportunity for a long-term relationship with the attractive young suitor she loves. This opportunity can only be reclaimed after the man falls victim to the deadly "Yellow Jack" epidemic, and she valiantly chooses to journey with him to the desolate island on which the infected are quarantined. In *Imitation of Life,* a mother struggles valiantly, until the moment of her death from an unspecified disease, to ensure the long-term well-being of her unappreciative daughter, as a means of correcting her failings in her socially expected maternal role. The mother's failings become evident in the degree of her suffering, which increases in direct proportion to the extent to which she loses control over her deviant offspring.

It is perhaps not at all surprising, therefore, that many AIDS movies are structured in ways similar to these melodramas, or that they deal with the social containment and eradication of otherness in similar ways. An outstanding example is provided by the 1996 AIDS movie *It's My Party*, in which Nick Stark (played by Eric Roberts), a gay man with AIDS, learns that he has only a few more days of conscious existence before the advanced lesions on his brain render him comatose. Refusing to meet his end blind, demented, and covered in his own excrement, Nick decides to throw a two-day party for his family members and closest friends before he takes his own life by drug overdose. Although his loved ones appear to desire a sentimental opportunity to grieve, Nick insists that they remain upbeat for the duration of the event, after which there will be no memorial service and no funeral. Similar to Judith Traherne in *Dark Victory*, therefore, Nick endeavors intentionally to sacrifice his own emotional needs to minimize the emotionality of his impending death for his closest loved ones. He tells jokes (e.g., a punch line points out that both soybeans and dildos are "meat substitutes") and alters song lyrics to match the occasion (e.g., emphasizing that it's his party and he'll "die" if he wants to). He presents expensive gifts to his family members and closest friends. He puts his concern for others ahead of concern for himself, asking a gay nephew to promise to engage always in safer sex; reminding a close friend to always make the choices in life that will ultimately make her happy; requesting that his Greek mother not wear black for the duration of her life as an indicator of mourning and loss; allowing the one great love of his life to repair their troubled relationship during his final opportunity to do so. And, when the moment finally arrives to take his own life, as his vision and memory continue to decline, Nick faces his end just as valiantly as Judith Traherne faced hers, in his bed, with memories of happier times running through his mind.

Several other AIDS movies assume similar narrative approaches. The gay architect Donald (played by Zeljko Ivanek) in *Our Sons* (1991), for example, chooses the ideal moment to pass away, after allowing his estranged mother to reenter his life, care for him, and comfort him in the night. The reformed intravenous drug user Linda (played by Mary-Louise Parker) in *A Place for Annie* (1994) termi-

nates her parental rights and goes off to die alone in an undisclosed
hospice, after ensuring that her infant daughter's needs will be
tended to by a loving family. The gay performance artist Charlie
(played by Robert Downey Jr.) in *One Night Stand* (1997) embraces
death only after he is certain that his best friend, Max (played by
Wesley Snipes), his own father, and various friends are adequately
prepared to thrive in their lives without him; throughout his physical decline, he maintains that his death is far harder for his friends
than it is for himself, and he remains fascinated by what may await
him in the next life.

What distinguishes these and other AIDS movies from traditional
melodramas, however, is that the otherness of their protagonists
derives primarily from their infection with HIV/AIDS—and frequently from their membership in traditionally peripheral groups
(such as gay men) as well—rather than from personality-based factors such as unrefined behavior (as in *Stella Dallas*) or an independent spirit (as in *Dark Victory*). From an ideological and representational standpoint, this distinction is quite noteworthy because it
suggests that individuals in such stigmatized social groups (or, at
the very least, those within the story world of AIDS movies) must
ultimately die to restore the patriarchal social order through the
eradication of their "deviant" otherness. Although Stella Dallas,
Judith Traherne, and other melodramatic protagonists ultimately are
capable of ridding themselves of their otherness, if ever they so
desire, simply by opting to conform to social expectations, protagonists in AIDS movies have no similar means (at present) by which
to rid themselves of the otherness of HIV/AIDS. Ideologically
speaking, therefore, unintended and undesirable social effects may
result when the narrative structures and representational approaches
to otherness common in melodramas—which strive, ultimately, to
marginalize any resistance to dominant ideologies (Byars, 1991,
p. 15)—surface in parallel ways in AIDS movies, in which they
serve to represent the otherness of individuals striving to overcome
infection with HIV/AIDS. Considering that the infected individuals
in AIDS movies typically die and frequently are members of stigmatized social groups, the implications of such a reality can be
startling.

Traditional melodramas focus on the protagonist as victim, and, for the most part, they strive to remain nostalgic, longing for a return to an ideal time of respectability that lacks antisocial and/or immoral behavior (Hayward, 1996, p. 205). In this sense, they are considered to represent a somewhat repressive type of movie, as they typically feature one-dimensional characters in plots in which good eventually triumphs over evil (Beaver, 1994, p. 230). As film scholar Richard Gollin explains, "Melodrama is a modern form of the old morality play in which long-tried virtue eventually subdues vice at great cost or is rescued from its helplessness before vice. The characters are all definable by their moral or social commitments even when these are mixed or ambivalent" (1992, p. 131). This means that human identity is treated by melodrama morally and affectively, with melodramas appealing to the viewer's emotions rather than to his or her reason or intellect (Lang, 1989, p. 49).

A typical feature of melodramas, therefore, is that the problems and social issues they address in the form of otherness are restricted to the level of individual characters rather than expanding the investigation of these issues and their causes to the larger social and political domain. Apparently, this individualized representational approach to otherness stems from the melodramatic intention to suggest that problems of otherness can indeed be resolved in some way, ultimately restoring the patriarchal social order. Such an approach becomes markedly more problematic, however, when it appears in similar ways in AIDS movies, at which point "another ideological spearhead is being launched against an enemy within" (Watney, 1996, p. 16). When this occurs, as AIDS activist Simon Watney has observed, the otherness that must be dealt with by the patriarchal social order becomes "not a virus which can and must be conquered but rather those who suffer from it, premised as the sexually promiscuous, and with them, by extension, all other enemies of 'the family,' the sacred and largely imaginary locus of neo-conservatism in all its variant forms and voices" (Ibid.).

Most commonly within AIDS movies, gay men are represented as the primary others who must be sacrificed to restore the patriarchal social order that existed prior to the discovery of HIV/AIDS; they are the sexually promiscuous "enemies" of both the family and the larger society to whom Watney refers. The resulting persistent link between gay men and AIDS in these movies, therefore—which is explored at length in Chapter 4 of this work— readily contributes to the social construction of a world in which differences in sexual orientation are devalued, and it perpetuates the pervasive ideologies of homophobia and heterosexism, to the detriment of all gay men in American society and their long-term social prospects.

OTHER FORMS OF OTHERNESS AND AIDS

Similar to melodramas and science fiction movies, AIDS movies influence the American social consciousness through the mediation of dominant ideologies and the social construction of attitudes and phenomena considered to be of particular significance during the period in which they are made. As the preceding discussion has shown, although the representational approaches pertaining to otherness in these three kinds of movies may be remarkably similar at times, the potential social effects of such approaches typically vary quite dramatically by movie type.

The present chapter has theorized the parallels between the representation of otherness in two specific kinds of offerings—science fiction movies and melodramas—and the representation of otherness in AIDS movies, to begin to define more fully the narrative form of the AIDS movie (with regard to its representational approaches to otherness) in relation to other kinds of movies that it resembles most closely, and with which many American movie viewers are likely to be more familiar. In the chapters that follow, three additional forms of otherness that are represented persistently in AIDS movies, and which stem from their representational parallels in science fiction movies, melodramas, and related cinematic offerings, are explored in depth: (1) the "us" versus "them" representation of innocent victims and guilty ones (as identified in this chapter's discussion of otherness and science fiction movies); (2) the typical representation of gay men as the "sacrificial other" in AIDS movies (as identified in this chapter's discussion of otherness and melodramas); and (3) the representational role of the city (versus the country) in American movies about HIV/AIDS.

Chapter 3

"Us" versus "Them": "Innocent Victims" and the Politics of Victim Blaming

In the 1994 AIDS movie *A Place for Annie,* Mary-Louise Parker plays Linda, a woman who contracts HIV/AIDS through intravenous drug use and gives birth to a daughter, Annie, who tests positive for HIV at birth and enters the world with a heroin addiction, as well. Linda disappears two days after Annie's birth, leaving her daughter in need of a foster home with loving parents who will not mind caring for an HIV-positive child. The odds of finding such a home appear slim, until Susan (played by Sissy Spacek), head nurse in a pediatric ward, takes to the child and decides to adopt her. Although warned by a social worker that she is setting herself up for a broken heart, Susan believes that Annie is worth the risk. She hires a nanny to care for Annie while she is at work, and her son pitches in occasionally to lend a helping hand. Annie's T-cell count remains below normal, and she experiences regular infections as she begins to grow, but otherwise she finds herself embraced by the warmth of a loving family.

During the first-anniversary celebration of Annie's status as a foster child, as the adoption paperwork makes its way through the system, Susan learns from the social worker that Linda wants Annie back. A custody hearing has already been arranged. Susan protests that Linda has no right to reclaim the child because not only did she abandon Annie but she is also a drug addict with AIDS. As such, Susan is saddened to learn that Linda is now free of drugs, and that her status as a person with AIDS is protected information under her right to privacy. She is also dismayed to learn that, as a foster mother who has not yet adopted the child, she has no legal rights of her own with regard to custody. Ultimately, the judge awards custody of Annie to Linda; Susan enacts a plan to have Linda move into her home, so she can still be with Annie. It is clear that Susan's actions stem from selfish motives rather than from a benevolent desire to assist the reformed drug abuser with AIDS. Before Linda moves in, for example, Susan reveals her contempt for the woman when she informs her that, in contrast to the reformed drug abuser who spent time hanging out on street corners injecting drugs with dirty needles, she herself has had to work continuously for everything she has.

Once moved in, Linda is revealed to be a bad mother (she loses her temper while playing with Annie) and a bad role model (she smokes constantly and almost burns down the house after her bed catches on fire). She also experiences chronic guilt about endangering the life of her child by giving birth to her. She apologizes to Annie for passing AIDS along to her, emphasizing that although she herself deserves the painful and lengthy demise that awaits her, Annie does not. All Linda wants is forgiveness for her drug-abusing past. But forgiveness can come only after doctors discover that Annie is no longer testing positive for the HIV antibodies and Linda terminates her parental rights. Before the movie concludes, a doctor informs Susan that there is no longer any reason to believe that Annie will not be able to live a long and completely healthy life. In other words, the innocent child is no longer destined to die from HIV/AIDS. In contrast, Linda's health is declining steadily, and she goes off to die alone. At movie's end, the viewer is left with two central questions: (1) Why does Annie suddenly receive a clean bill of health while there is no hope left for Linda? (2) Why is the death of a heterosexual woman who became infected with HIV/AIDS through intravenous drug use not worthy of being portrayed on-screen, and how might this differ if the narrative involved the impending death of a heterosexual woman who became infected through heterosexual sexual activity?

"VILLAINS" AND "INNOCENT VICTIMS"

Certainly, a regular form of otherness contained in AIDS movies involves the status of "innocent victims," which results from the

social construction of certain kinds of people with AIDS as victim-
izers of "innocent bystanders" (Erni, 1994, p. 51). This construction
creates and reinforces the harmful notion that Americans fit into
two broad categories in relation to HIV/AIDS: (1) the "us"/the
"normal"/the "general population," containing "innocent" individuals threatened not by their own risk behaviors but by individuals in
the "other" category; and (2) the "them"/"villains" in this health
crisis, containing those who are "guilty," who are to be blamed for
AIDS, who threaten the health of innocent others, and who are
perceived neither as experiencing human suffering nor deserving of
attention and sympathy but rather as the source of threat to members of the general population (Croteau and Morgan, 1989, p. 87;
Gross, 1994, p. 147).

The resulting "us" versus "them" dichotomy has been continually communicated in American society by various social actors, such
as in 1985, when CBS anchor Dan Rather introduced a story about
AIDS by emphasizing that scientists now realize the disease can
strike within the bounds of "respectable society" and that it does not
result solely from the "immoral" actions of intravenous drug users
and gay men (Cook and Colby, 1992, p. 99). That same year, then-
Secretary of Health and Human Services Margaret Heckler an-
nounced that AIDS must be conquered before it becomes an over-
whelming problem by affecting members of the "heterosexual
population" and the "general population" (Shilts, 1987, p. 554). As
counselor James Croteau and sociologist Susanne Morgan point
out, with this statement, Heckler "showed both high regard for the us
or the general population and a clear callousness toward the other"
(1989, p. 87), which consists primarily of gay men and intravenous
drug users—members of two large groups in American society who
have traditionally evoked social discomfort and/or social antago-
nism (Pryor and Reeder, 1993, p. vii). President Ronald Reagan
showed similar callousness in his 1987 address to the American
Foundation for AIDS Research (AmFAR) when he explained that
human decency requires all individuals who believe they may be
carriers of AIDS to be tested because "innocent people" are now
being infected with HIV, and some of them will advance to full-
blown AIDS and die (Nelson, 1999, p. 57).

Statements such as these leave audience members with the unfortunate impression that many of those Americans who became infected with or died from HIV/AIDS during the pandemic's early years were not innocent or, at the very least, that they were responsible for their illness (Nelson, 1999, p. 57). In addition, they suggest that the effects of HIV/AIDS are problematic only to those Americans who are outside the boundaries of what the most influential social actors have defined to be the problem (Cadwell, 1991, p. 239).

Physicians asked to complete the sentence "AIDS is like . . ." have frequently mentioned harmful metaphors such as "the wrath of God," "a plague brought to us by a minority of aberrant individuals," and "poetic justice, almost" (Pryor and Reeder, 1993, p. 279). Because the social construction of AIDS initially linked the pandemic primarily with gay men and intravenous drug users, responsibility for AIDS has readily been attributed to their "deviant" behavior and marginalized status rather than to infection by a deleterious microorganism (Wright, 1997, p. 75). Sociologist Eric Wright emphasizes that the most important effect of AIDS being associated with members of these marginal and deviant groups is that an us-versus-them ideology makes it easier for members of the general population to separate themselves from the people who have the disease and, indirectly, from the disease itself (Ibid.).

In this regard, the general population is presumed to be heterosexual, middle to upper class, family centered, non-pleasure seeking, and unaddicted (seemingly in apparent contrast to gay men and drug abusers), as well as the repository of everything individuals enjoy claiming for themselves yet denying to others (Yep and Pietri, 1999, p. 200; Grover, 1987, p. 24). Wright explains that an important way for the general population to generate a sense of distance from the pandemic is by "blaming the victim" of the disease, such as by attributing the cause of contracting HIV/AIDS entirely to specific deviant behaviors (primarily homosexual sexual activity and intravenous drug use) and characterizing it as deserved punishment for those who are unable or unwilling to control their immoral behavior (Wright, 1997, p. 75; Slagle, 1999, p. 93). Victim blaming in relation to members of deviant groups, therefore, serves as a strategy by which to make something that is incomprehensible somehow explainable and, thereby, seemingly controllable, as well as a means by which to locate the locus of risk outside of oneself and in "the other" (Cadwell, 1991, p. 240).

Additional explanations employed to achieve a similar distancing effect include the arguments that gay men and intravenous drug users must endure HIV/AIDS as punishment by God for their sins or to compensate for the general social and moral decay in American society (Wright, 1997, p. 75). Such distancing strategies tend to overlook the realities of the worldwide pandemic, in which AIDS is overwhelmingly the result of heterosexual sexual transmission and not necessarily the result of deviant behaviors (Herek and Glunt, 1988, p. 888). At the same time, they position certain members of American society—infants, children, hemophiliacs, blood transfusion recipients, heterosexuals—to be considered "innocent victims" rather than "deviant villains" if ever they contract HIV/AIDS themselves.

Throughout the ages, humans have tended to distort reality and construct experiences that enable them to avoid, to as great an extent as possible, a fundamental anxiety about death from infectious diseases by linguistically managing the ambiguity and uncertainty surrounding such diseases to reduce panic (Clark, 1999, p. 19). As Susan Sontag has noted, every feared epidemic disease, past and present, has generated a preoccupying distinction between the putative carriers of that disease and those defined as the general population, with the carriers being viewed as morally polluted and the disease serving as a metaphor for morality (1989, p. 115). The resulting social consequences of reactions to infectious diseases are determined, in large part, however, by the number of individuals they affect. As sociologist William Rushing explains:

> When an infectious disease affects only one individual or a few persons, the sociological significance of the fear of contagion is limited to its effects on those who are sick. If the disease is widespread and becomes an epidemic, the fear of contagion and its social effects are more widespread. Then, according to historical studies, a "traumatic shock on a societal level" may occur, accompanied by extreme collective actions: massive migration; desertion, persecution, punitive quarantines, and os-

tracism of the sick; riots; and accusations that certain groups
cause the disease (scapegoating). . . . (1995, p. 130)

Rushing points out that such extreme reactions occur in epidemics whenever four conditions are met: (1) the disease is quite lethal;
(2) the disease emerges (or at least appears to emerge) suddenly;
(3) the death rate rises quickly, to the point that many believe the
general population is at serious risk of contracting the disease; and
(4) there does not appear to be a ready explanation for the disease
(1995, p. 130). As such, because the cause of Spanish flu was
known, there was little in the way of mass panic, extreme collective
reactions, or scapegoating during the months in 1918 and 1919
when the Spanish influenza epidemic killed approximately 20 mil-
lion people around the world (Ibid.). In contrast, AIDS, during the
early years of the pandemic—similar to the Black Death in Europe
during the Middle Ages and the cholera epidemics in Europe and
the United States during the 1800s—met all four of the conditions
identified by Rushing, resulting in social hysteria and the moralistic
scapegoating of certain types of individuals as the causes of HIV/
AIDS. Because the virus that causes AIDS was not discovered until
1984, three years after the epidemic began, and the mode of its
transmission was not clarified until some time later, the association
of HIV/AIDS with the deviance of gay men and intravenous drug
users seized the American consciousness early on and has persisted
to this day (Ibid., p. 170).

The groups selected to serve as scapegoats for infectious epidemics tend to be those against whom members of dominant social
groups harbor hostility or suspicion and regard as social outcasts
(Rushing, 1995, p. 166); thus, the resulting classifications of innocent victims and guilty ones reflect the beliefs, stereotypes, and
political biases of the culture and era in which they are socially
constructed (Cadwell, 1991, p. 240). To effectively create one or
more scapegoats, influential social actors must, in some way, per-
suade others that such scapegoats are "worthy" of sacrifice (Slagle,
1999, p. 100). By initially constructing HIV/AIDS as a disease transmitted almost exclusively through anal intercourse between gay
men and through intravenous drug injection, fears of contagion
among members of the general population were reduced consider-

ably during the early years of the pandemic, and those fears have generally remained at relatively low levels since, despite the changing demographics of the pandemic. With regard to the AIDS movie *A Place for Annie,* therefore, this discussion helps to explain why the innocent victim, Annie, unexpectedly receives a clean bill of health at movie's end while the guilty and deviant (albeit reformed) intravenous drug user, Linda, must die alone, with her death not being worthy of portrayal on-screen.

THE PROCESS OF VICTIM BLAMING IN AIDS MOVIES

The social-construction perspective maintains that individuals react to a particular disease according to the way in which it has been defined for them, regardless of the scientific validity of that definition (Rushing, 1995, p. 163). Frequently, the definition of a disease reflects social and cultural conditions more than biological ones (Ibid.). With regard to HIV/AIDS, specifically, part of this definition includes a "victim continuum" for categorizing people with AIDS, which distinguishes innocent victims from guilty ones and acknowledges differential degrees of innocence/guilt (McKinney and Pepper, 1999, p. 87). The existence of this continuum was perhaps best reflected in the debate over the ultimate title of the 1989 AIDS movie *The Littlest Victims,* which was changed from *The Most Innocent Victims* at the last minute under pressure from gay activists and AIDS activists (Goldstein, 1991, p. 28). On one end of this continuum are completely innocent victims who contract HIV/AIDS entirely through the fault of others, such as infants born to infected mothers, hemophiliacs, and blood transfusion recipients. On the other end of this continuum are guilty victims who contract HIV/AIDS through their intentional pursuit of "deviant" and "immoral" behaviors, such as gay men and intravenous drug users. Somewhere in between fall heterosexual men and women who contract HIV/AIDS as a result of their own sexual activities, but do not engage in "deviant" practices, such as anal intercourse or drug injection.

These distinctions are noteworthy because sympathy at the societal level is typically garnered only for those who become infected with HIV/AIDS through absolutely no fault of their own (Netzham-

mer and Shamp, 1994, p. 98), as well as for those generally monogamous, not-too-promiscuous heterosexuals who contract HIV/AIDS
as a result of heterosexual sexual activity; these individuals are therefore considered to be relatively innocent victims. Such distinctions
are also relevant to the present discussion because they serve to
explain more fully why the character, Linda, in *A Place for Annie*
must die alone, excluded from the sympathy and support of surrounding others, whereas Robin (also played by Mary-Louise Parker), in the 1994 AIDS movie *Boys on the Side*, who contracted
HIV/AIDS as a result of heterosexual sex with a bartender, is representationally permitted to remain in the company of loving and
caring others until she ultimately succumbs to the disease.

Social information about this victim continuum is communicated
to viewers of AIDS movies in various ways. Many movies provide
such information blatantly in the form of character dialogue, such
as when the character Lady Marmalade (played by Michael Lynch)
in *Chocolate Babies* (1996) explains that innocent victims get "Mag-
ic Johnson disease" or "Ryan White's disease," whereas gay men and
intravenous drug users get AIDS, and the government doesn't care at
all about the people who get AIDS. Similarly, a (presumably heterosexual, non-drug-injecting) television newscaster in the 1986 AIDS
movie *As Is* explains how fortunate it is that AIDS has largely been
confined to members of high-risk groups and has only rarely affected innocent Americans "like you and me." In another example,
while attempting to make a videotape for his estranged father, gay
character Nick (played by Steve Buscemi), in the 1986 AIDS movie
Parting Glances, finds it necessary to explain that he stopped engaging in casual sexual encounters when he learned of AIDS, and
that he didn't have that many of them before that point, so his father
should not go around saying that contracting AIDS was his own
fault because it was not. The character Luanne (played by Ann-
Margret) in the 1991 AIDS movie *Our Sons* explains that her gay
son's battle with AIDS is "God's will." A homophobic shopper in
the 1992 AIDS movie *The Living End* explains that, contrary to
popular belief, the acronym AIDS really stands for "Adios, Infected
Dick-Suckers." The promiscuous party animal Tracy, in the 1992
AIDS movie *Something to Live For: The Alison Gertz Story,* insists
that she, rather than Alison, deserves to be dying of AIDS because it

was she who was partying wildly and sleeping with numerous men, whereas Alison cheated on her boyfriend only once, during a one-night stand. The character John Jeckyll (played by John Glover) in the 1997 AIDS movie *Love! Valour! Compassion!,* during a moment of anger, wishes AIDS on another gay man who has offended him because he feels that the man's offensive actions deserve harsh punishment, emphasizing that he hopes the man dies from the condition. Exchanges of dialogue such as these efficiently perpetuate the us-versus-them dichotomy with regard to "innocent" and "guilty" people with AIDS.

Less blatantly, some AIDS movies are constructed in such a way as to imply that AIDS is the deserved punishment for individuals who choose to violate widely shared social and moral norms. The narrative of the 1992 AIDS movie *Citizen Cohn,* for example, is constructed as an extended trial of the closeted homosexual and vindictive communist headhunter Roy Cohn by the ghosts of victims he has wronged in his past, with Cohn's ultimate death from AIDS representing "just punishment" for his various offenses. Similarly, the only heterosexual male with AIDS represented in the 1985 AIDS movie *An Early Frost* will be forced to face a prolonged, painful death as a result of his having unprotected sex with a female prostitute rather than with a more upstanding heterosexual female. The two AIDS characters in the 1995 AIDS movie *The Immortals,* one a gay man and the other a heterosexual intravenous drug user, are recruited to take part in an elaborate crime exclusively because they are socially undesirable, "dispensable" individuals. For these characters and others similar to them, AIDS is depicted as the most appropriate form of punishment for their social and moral transgressions, a punishment deserved by those who freely choose to be irresponsible and to deviate from society's prescribed rules (McKinney and Pepper, 1999, p. 90).

In striking contrast to these examples is the representation of AIDS with regard to innocent victims, which is explained by a reverend in *The Ryan White Story* (1989) to be the awesome and wonderful mystery of God's will and God's love. Relatedly, despite all of the deviance and moral transgressions present in the 1995 AIDS movie *Kids*—including (but certainly not limited to) instances of extreme violence, casual sex, and excessive drug abuse—the character Jennie (played by Chloe Sevigny) is still represented to be a relatively innocent victim after she loses her virginity to Telly, thereby contracting HIV through unprotected heterosexual sex.

Perhaps least blatantly of all, AIDS movies specifically about innocent victims communicate social information about the AIDS victim continuum by unnecessarily introducing the topic of homosexuality into their narratives. The two most prominent examples of this process occur in *The Ryan White Story* (1989) and *The Cure* (1995). *The Ryan White Story* is based on real-life experiences of the young hemophiliac who became infected with HIV in the mid-1980s and who (along with his family members) fought for the right of a person with AIDS to continue attending classes in a public school. Perhaps to solidify Ryan's status as a truly innocent victim within this movie, the narrative contains a brief scene in which two boys playing outside a church shout names at the youth, specifically "Homo!" and "Queer!"; another brief scene presents a young girl informing Ryan's sister that her brother said Ryan is a "faggot" because he has contracted AIDS. The unnecessary introduction of derogatory terms pertaining to homosexuality in these instances suggests to the viewer that there are indeed villains in the health crisis that Ryan is confronting, and that those villains, specifically, are gay men. Similarly, *The Cure*, a fictional narrative about an eleven-year-old boy who contracted HIV/AIDS through a blood transfusion shortly after he was born, unnecessarily contains a rather lengthy scene in which this innocent victim and his male friend are accosted by other boys in their neighborhood and referred to as "faggots" because one of them is infected with AIDS and they have crossed into a "no-homo zone." Again, in this instance, the topic of homosexuality is introduced into a narrative that could proceed quite logically and effectively without it, ultimately reinforcing notions of gay men as guilty victims and others as innocent ones.

An exchange of dialogue from the 1993 AIDS movie *Grief,* between a gay man and his two heterosexual female co-workers in the entertainment industry, effectively encapsulates the issues central to the process of victim blaming in AIDS movies. When asked whatever became of an AIDS script that had been worked on for several weeks, the gay writer explains that, although he wanted the central character with AIDS to be an "innocent" gay man, others insisted that the character be an "innocent" seven year old, so he abandoned the project. He adds that his previous attempt to compose a serious gay AIDS story line that did not place blame on the character contracting HIV/AIDS was also rejected by the powers-that-be at the production company, who instead turned the character into a sex-crazed psychopath. In other words, the socially constructed discourse surrounding HIV/AIDS positions the self (a member of the general population) in extreme opposition to the other (a social deviant, such as a gay man, an intravenous drug user, or even a psychopath), thereby creating and maintaining the illusion of a safe distance between individuals presumed to be infected with HIV/AIDS and everybody else (Yep and Pietri, 1999, p. 200).

As we begin a new millennium, what AIDS movies and American society need to do now is to shift their focus away from the social constructions of "innocent" and "guilty" victims and toward the phenomenon of "invisible" victims, those many members of the general population who inaccurately believe that they are shielded from infection with HIV/AIDS by virtue of their nondeviant social identity. The words spoken by Doreen Millman in 1996, at the Eleventh International Conference on AIDS, ring especially true in this regard. Acknowledging that audience members would be wondering how she, a sixty-three-year-old grandmother, became infected with HIV, Millman pointed out that the answer was quite simple: it really does not matter (Millman, 1996, p. 1). Everyone needs accurate information about the current realities of the AIDS pandemic that traditional us-versus-them representations, no matter how comforting to the non-drug-injecting heterosexual majority they may be, simply do not provide. The most promising alternative to AIDS narratives involving victim blaming lies in the regular creation and dissemination of prosocial narratives about caring for others in their times of need, despite individual differences and despite the means by which they have contracted HIV/AIDS.

Chapter 4

Gay Men As "The (Primary) Other" in the AIDS Movie

In 1981, physicians in California and New York began identifying what would later become known as America's first AIDS cases. More specifically, they began diagnosing the occurrence of two diseases—a rare form of cancer called Kaposi's sarcoma (KS) and a rare form of pneumonia (PCP) caused by the *Pneumocystis carinii* organism—in gay male patients with mysteriously ravaged immune systems (Pryor and Reeder, 1993, p. 269). In June and July 1981, the Centers for Disease Control (CDC) reported such findings pertaining to thirty-one young gay men; statistics released soon thereafter similarly revealed a high concentration of PCP, KS, and related opportunistic afflictions among gay males (Rushing, 1995, p. 15). As a result, medical authorities officially recognized the demographic characteristic these patients had in common when labeling their resulting condition GRID, which stood for "gay-related immune deficiency," even though the first heterosexual patients with similar health conditions, including the first women, were reported by the CDC that same summer (Padgug and Oppenheimer, 1992, p. 253). By the time the term *AIDS* was adopted by the CDC in 1982, the disease had been solidly constructed in the minds of Americans as a "gay disease," even though studies had identified nongay individuals with AIDS from the pandemic's early days (Ibid.).

Stories associating gay men with AIDS appeared in American news media in 1982; many suggested that the behaviors of gay men were directly responsible for the disease and that it was directly related to their deviant sexual practices (Cook and Colby, 1992, p. 93; Rushing, 1995, p. 99). Although CDC information regularly revealed the spread of AIDS beyond gay men throughout 1982 and 1983 (Cook and Colby, 1992, p. 93), nearly all mass media attention paid to gay men by 1983 involved AIDS-related stories (Gross, 1994, p. 145), and media professionals remained reluctant to stray from the view of AIDS as a gay disease (Slagle, 1999, p. 95). In a NBC news report on August 17, 1984, a story about the isolation of the virus that causes AIDS, for example, emphasized that although scientists and researchers do not know for certain what causes AIDS, they know that it primarily attacks and kills gay men (Cook and Colby, 1992, p. 104). Lifestyle reporters at the time commonly interrogated gay men with AIDS about their lives and lifestyles; their "unspoken clauses rendered the answers ambiguous enough to erase anything positive an individual might try to say. 'How do you feel now (read: that your "lifestyle" has betrayed you)?' 'Was it (sex) worth it (death)?' " (Patton, 1990, p. 25). As AIDS activist Cindy Patton has observed, in human interest stories during the years 1981 to 1985, which were aimed at a general public that wanted to feel safe from the pandemic, the gay man with AIDS stood in for "Anglo-American culture which, at the edge of the twenty-first century, is still unable to separate its fear of sexuality from the vicissitudes of a little understood virus" (Ibid.).

Considering the socially constructed environment within which AIDS seized the anxious imagination of the American public, it is perhaps unsurprising that the stigma of AIDS found itself inextricably linked to the stigma of homosexuality from the onset of the pandemic (Clark, 1999, p. 9). Despite the changing demographics of the AIDS pandemic, early conceptualizations of AIDS as a "gay disease" and "gay plague" have persisted, with fear of AIDS representing for many Americans "a more strident articulation of fear of gays" (Cadwell, 1991, p. 240). As clinical social worker Steve Cadwell explains, "Rooting out the 'abnormal' homosexual was replaced by a shrill cry to rid the society of the cancerous growth of AIDS. The object of discrimination remained the same—gay men" (Ibid.). In other words, gay men who were already stigmatized as deviant were further stigmatized as lethally contagious; as such, they were socially constructed as posing a greater threat to America's heterosexist social order than ever before (Ibid., p. 237).

The initial construction of AIDS, with its emphasis on a particular (gay) lifestyle rather than on particular (risk) behaviors, thereby singled out the gay male other as the primary threat to the general population. For many Americans, the identification of gay men as members of a high-risk group falsely implied that all gay men were inherently at greater risk of contracting HIV/AIDS than were members of other groups and that all gay men regularly engaged in high-risk behaviors (Rushing, 1995, p. 16). In the process, the positive representational strides achieved by gay men in the late 1970s and early 1980s suffered serious setbacks, as AIDS became representationally linked to them, and the term *gay*, which had been wrenched away from the earlier pejorative discourse of homosexuality, was reloaded with stereotypical connotations of effeminacy, contagion, and degeneracy (Watney, 1996, p. 18).

The social construction of AIDS in relation to gay men effectively limited the space for alternative imaginings of the pandemic and those affected by it (Erni, 1994, p. 50). Despite ongoing efforts by various social actors, this initial perception of AIDS as a gay disease has proven difficult to overcome (Slagle, 1999, p. 93). It is perhaps unsurprising as well, therefore, that the central characters with HIV/AIDS in the earliest AIDS movies—including *An Early Frost* (1985), *Buddies* (1985), *As Is* (1986), and *Parting Glances* (1986)—were all represented to be gay men. What is a bit more surprising, however, is the number of AIDS movies that have continued to reinforce the persistent link between gay men and AIDS over the past two decades. Of the thirty-two AIDS movies analyzed in this study, for example, 75 percent of them (n = 24) contain at least one gay male character with HIV/AIDS. In addition, of the six most recent AIDS movies analyzed —*Breaking the Surface: The Greg Louganis Story* (1996), *It's My Party* (1996), *In the Gloaming* (1997), *Love! Valour! Compassion!* (1997), *One Night Stand* (1997), and *Gia* (1998)— all but one feature a gay male as the central character with HIV/AIDS. This suggests that the construction of AIDS as a "gay disease" has only occasionally been challenged in AIDS movies over time, ultimately reinforcing that construction. As the discussion in this chapter reveals, such a reality has been problematic for gay men in American society as well as members of various other demographic groups.

THE PERSISTENT REPRESENTATIONAL
LINK BETWEEN GAY MEN AND AIDS:
OPPORTUNITIES, SHORTCOMINGS,
AND CONSEQUENCES FOR GAY MALES

As explained in Chapter 1 (and consistent with previous research efforts on the representation of AIDS in American media offerings), the term *AIDS* is being used in this study to refer both to the condition of infection with HIV and to the condition of experiencing the multiple disease pattern referred to as acquired immunodeficiency syndrome. The coding scheme for the content-analytic portion of this study, therefore, specified that for any character in an AIDS movie to be considered an "AIDS character," it must be evident from the movie's manifest content that (1) the character is indeed infected with HIV or AIDS and (2) the character has either a name (first name and/or last name) and/or at least one line of dialogue. The former criterion was included to ensure that only characters explicitly identified as having HIV or AIDS would be coded as "AIDS characters"; the latter criterion was included as a means of distinguishing characters from extras. As such, a character named Doug at a doctor's office who is informed that he has tested positive for HIV would be coded as an AIDS character in this study. In contrast, a character at a doctor's office who reads an informational brochure about AIDS while sitting in the waiting room would not be coded as an AIDS character in this study because it is unclear whether this character is actually infected with HIV or AIDS, as well as because the character has no name and no lines of dialogue, suggesting that he or she is simply an extra in the movie rather than a major or minor character. The consistent application of these coding criteria served to ensure that the manifest contents of the AIDS movies in this study were analyzed systematically (according to explicit and consistently applied rules) and objectively (if replicated by another researcher, the analysis should yield the same results) (Wimmer and Dominick, 1991, pp. 157-158).

Application of this coding scheme yielded a total of seventy-six AIDS characters in the thirty-two AIDS movies analyzed. The clear majority of these AIDS characters, 68.4 percent (n = 52), are gay males, compared with 13.2 percent (n = 10) heterosexual females,

11.8 percent (n = 9) heterosexual males, and 1.3 percent (n = 1) bisexual females. It was not possible to accurately determine the manifest sexual orientation of an additional 5.3 percent (n = 4) of AIDS characters in these movies, all of whom were male. These movies included no lesbian or bisexual male characters with AIDS.

Although the primary reliance on representing gay men as individuals with AIDS in these movies has been unfortunate for the social construction of the pandemic, it nevertheless provided numerous additional opportunities for the representation of gay men on American movie theater and television screens. As such, the representations of gay men in AIDS movies have retained the potential to shape the way that Americans come to understand the phenomenon of homosexuality and to influence the relationships within and among various social groups in American society. In other words, even though the persistent representational link between gay men and AIDS in these movies has been harmful to the resulting social construction of the pandemic, these movies still offer numerous unique opportunities for the representation of various members of the gay community because they regularly feature the gay male lovers and close gay friends of characters with HIV/AIDS. They offer significant possibilities for altering and expanding the commonly accepted ways in which nongays perceive and discuss the status of gay men and their lived realities in modern American society. So just what sorts of messages about gay men are commonly communicated in these movies? How positively or negatively are members of the gay community represented in them overall?

"Representation is a very different notion from that of reflection," explains cultural studies scholar Stuart Hall. "It implies the active work of selecting and presenting, of structuring and shaping: not merely the transmitting of already-existing meaning, but the more active labor of making things mean" (1982, p. 64). Accordingly, the representation of gay men in AIDS movies has provided ideological guidance to American audience members about gay males and their lived realities, stemming from the codes, conventions, symbols, themes, and visuals the makers of these movies have chosen to include. Because many heterosexual Americans do not (knowingly) interact with gay men on a regular basis, media representations of gay men can be quite influential in the formation and modification of their perceptions. As media scholar Larry Gross has noted:

> The contributions of the mass media are likely to be especially powerful in cultivating images of groups and phenomena about which there is little firsthand opportunity for learning, particularly when such images are not contradicted by other established beliefs and ideologies. By definition, portrayals of minority groups and "deviants" will be relatively distant from the real lives of the large majority of viewers. Thus, in the case of . . . gay men we might reasonably expect that the media play a major role in shaping the images held by society, including in many cases by gay people ourselves. (1994, p. 144)

As such, the regular representation of gay men in AIDS movies has contributed significantly to "the 'coming out' of the gay community" because it results from "the deliberate desire to tear away the curtain of invisibility that had hitherto enveloped it" (Padgug and Oppenheimer, 1992, p. 251). However, as Larry Gross has cautioned, when groups such as gay men actually do attain regular media visibility, the manner of their representation typically reflects the perceptions, biases, and interests of the primarily white, heterosexual, middle-aged, and middle- to upper-middle-class social actors who most significantly define the American social agenda (1994, p. 143). With regard to the majority of AIDS movies analyzed in this study, which were produced for mainstream audiences, this suggests that the ideological guidance provided to viewers emerges out of representational power relations that place the majority of control over representation in the hands of rich, white, heterosexual males (Dyer, 1993, p. 2). Accordingly, the social construction of AIDS in such narrative works also serves, as well as masks, relations of power in American society (Fee and Fox, 1992, p. 17). A smaller number of AIDS movies analyzed here, however, were created under the guidance of gay male directors and/or targeted largely to gay male viewers in the form of independent theatrical releases, opening up a space for differential representations of gay men that may more accurately portray realities associated with the gay male experience in modern American society.

The most common representation of gay men in AIDS movies portrays gay men as embarrassments to their parents, particularly their fathers, with whom they have especially strained (or even nonexistent) relationships after they reveal their homosexuality. In the 1985 AIDS movie *An Early Frost,* for example, lawyer Michael (played by Aidan Quinn) is almost physically assaulted by his father when he reveals to his parents that he is gay. The man raises a fist to strike his son but is stopped by Michael's mother. Thereafter, the father who had always been so proud of his son's athletic and professional accomplishments grows distant and refers to Michael as a "stranger." Although Michael's mother strives to be supportive and desires to care for her HIV-positive child, his father insists that Michael can get care from his "own kind." In the 1995 AIDS movie *World and Time Enough,* found-object collector Joey (played by Gregory Giles) brings home his monogamous gay lover to meet his parents on Thanksgiving and is ordered to leave the house by his father, who calls his son a pervert and says he wishes the young man had never been born. Years later within the movie, Joey still runs out the back door of his parents' home whenever his father returns from work while he is visiting his mother. In the 1996 AIDS movie *It's My Party,* architect Nick Stark (played by Eric Roberts) misses out on a relationship with his father for two decades because the father is so ashamed that his son is gay. Similar examples can be found in several other AIDS movies, including *Parting Glances* (1986), *Breaking the Surface: The Greg Louganis Story* (1996), *In the Gloaming* (1997), and *One Night Stand* (1997).

In AIDS movies in which fathers are entirely absent and single mothers have raised their gay sons alone, it is often the mother who is ashamed of her son's homosexuality and who experiences a strained or nonexistent relationship with that son. In the 1991 AIDS movie *Our Sons,* for instance, the twenty-eight-year-old architect Donald (played by Zeljko Ivanek) has not spoken to his mother in years because, as Donald's lover explains, the woman's response to her son's sexual orientation was far less than enlightened. Donald's mother kicked her son out of the house when he was seventeen years old after learning that he was gay, because she hates what he is. She constantly dwells on the distinction between a man being gay or "being normal," and she finds it impossible to believe that any mother would not be extremely bothered by a son being "one of them." Similarly, in the 1996 AIDS movie *Chocolate Babies*, the warm relationship between the young AIDS activist Sam (played by Jon Lee) and his mother becomes quite strained after he reveals his homosexuality to her: she responds by referring to his gay friends as "freaks" and "faggots," resenting them for turning her son into a "fag."

Such representations contribute to the social construction of a society in which differences are devalued, and they also perpetuate heterosexism, the ideological system that "denies, denigrates, and stigmatizes any nonheterosexual form of behavior, identity, relationship, or community" (Herek, 1992, p. 89), and that stereotypes gay men as being effeminate, passive, and deviant.

Another very common representation of gay men in AIDS movies portrays them as sexually promiscuous individuals who irresponsibly put others at risk of contracting HIV/AIDS. In the 1985 AIDS movie *An Early Frost*, Michael learns that his lover, Peter (played by D. W. Moffett), slept with random men he met in gay bars and at a bathhouse when Michael became too consumed with his work to fulfill his sexual needs. In the 1986 AIDS movie *As Is*, the short-story author Rich (played by Robert Carradine) cruises bars regularly and picks up all kinds of guys, from conservative men to leather men. In the 1992 AIDS movie *The Living End*, the handsome and HIV-positive drifter Luke (played by Mike Dytri) engages in kinky sex with one man who picked him up while hitchhiking and then seduces another gay man just a few hours later. In the 1994 AIDS movie *Under Heat*, thirtysomething Dean (played by Eric Swanson) returns home to tell his mother and brother that he is HIV positive and becomes instantly attracted to Simon (played by David Conrad), the much younger male who mows his mother's lawn. The night after the two first meet, Simon climbs through Dean's bedroom window unexpectedly, and they immediately have sex. In the 1996 AIDS movie *Chocolate Babies*, the members of the self-proclaimed band of "raging, atheist, meat-eating, HIV-positive terrorists" engage regularly in unprotected sex and enjoy cutting their hands and smearing their infected blood on conservative politicians. Additional examples of gay men represented as irresponsibly promiscuous individuals can be found in

AIDS movies such as *Parting Glances* (1986), *Jerker* (1991), *And the Band Played On* (1993), *Grief* (1993), *World and Time Enough* (1995), and *Breaking the Surface: The Greg Louganis Story* (1996).

Although the regular representation of promiscuous gay men is somewhat understandable in movies set during the earliest years of the AIDS pandemic, this representational approach remains quite common in AIDS movies set in the late 1980s, and in the 1990s as well. As such, these negative representations can readily contribute to decreased levels of social tolerance for gay men in American society as well as increased levels of homophobia because they suggest that homosexuality no longer only threatens norms; it also threatens lives (Netzhammer and Shamp, 1994, p. 103). In addition, such representations serve to solidify the inaccurate perceptions that all gay men engage regularly in high-risk sexual behaviors and that they all partake of a "repulsive, deviant lifestyle" (Erni, 1994, p. 109).

In their discussion of what it takes to ensure that representations of gay men which are intended to be positive actually achieve that goal, counselor James Croteau and sociologist Susanne Morgan explain that representations of gay male sexuality should avoid implying the superiority of heterosexual expression by withholding presentations of the full range of choices available in homosexual expression (1989, p. 88). It is somewhat surprising to note, therefore, that almost all AIDS movies targeted to mainstream audiences handle presentations of gay male sexuality with kid gloves. In their assessment of television movies during the first decade of AIDS, scholars Frank Pilipp and Charles Shull conclude that AIDS movies only minimally focus on the pandemic as it is experienced by gay men, with modes of contraction and prevention only rarely being addressed and sex between men never being discussed (1993, p. 20).

During the preproduction stage of NBC's 1985 AIDS movie *An Early Frost*, for example, the network's broadcast standards department was far more concerned about the movie's treatment of homosexuality than with its treatment of AIDS because the network was fearful of including anything in the script that could be seen as condoning homosexuality (Farber, 1985, p. 23). AIDS activist Simon Watney has referred to this process as "institutional censorship," which he feels "guarantees a constant muting effect throughout the representation of AIDS [that is] rationalized as 'professionalism,' and justified in commercial terms of ratings" (1996, p. 112). As such, Watney considers *An Early Frost* to be a severely compromised creation that caters to relatively simplistic conceptions of network responsibility to the majority public (Ibid.). Film scholar Darrel Yates Rist has extended this line of argument by explaining that, although *An Early Frost* did not necessarily need to show two men French-kissing on-screen in prime time, the movie did need to somehow indicate that gay characters Michael and Peter were more than just roommates or best friends during their private moments together (Ibid., p. 113).

Certainly, the squeamish treatment of gay male sexuality that began in *An Early Frost* has persisted in the majority of mainstream AIDS movies since. Although producers' fears that media content cannot be as graphic when it is intended for mass audiences are somewhat understandable from a business standpoint (Farber, 1985, p. 23), the temptation to make mainstream movies about AIDS without making movies about homosexuality is quite similar to the temptation media professionals yielded to early in the pandemic, when they opted to ignore AIDS as legitimate news because it appeared to affect only gay men, with apparently far-reaching social consequences (Cook and Colby, 1992, p. 113).

Perhaps the most outstanding example of this process occurs in the 1993 AIDS movie *Philadelphia,* which is widely regarded as mainstream Hollywood's first all-star movie about AIDS. Although the presence of popular actors Tom Hanks and Antonio Banderas, playing gay lovers Andrew Beckett and Miguel Alvarez, was intended to lure hordes of straight viewers to sit through an AIDS movie and to make their introduction to the realities of modern gay life palatable, the representation of gay male sexuality in this offering remains largely at the level of television-movie-like touches. It is clear from the manifest content of this movie that Miguel cares deeply for Andrew, as he runs all the way to the hospital to which Andrew has been admitted, keeps records of Andrew's medical visits, and regrets that his and Andrew's days together are too quickly coming to an end. However, with the exception of one scene in which Andrew and Miguel slow dance at a costume party alongside Andrew's straight attorney and the attorney's wife, little within the movie's content reveals that these gay men are actually sexually involved lovers rather than simply very close roommates or best friends. Even when they are alone in Andrew's hospital room and Andrew reveals that he is ready to die, Miguel's greatest display of intimacy during his final moments with the character superficially encoded to be the great love of his life involves his kissing a couple of Andrew's fingers and then holding Andrew's hand. Such kid-glove treatment of gay male sexuality is especially suspect in a movie that contains lines of dialogue from one of its major characters, Andrew's homophobic attorney Joe Miller (played by Denzel Washington), emphasizing that everybody today is thinking about sexual orientation—about who does what to whom and how—and that the time has come to bring the topic out of the closet.

Similar repressive representations of gay male sexuality can readily be found in other AIDS movies. For example, in *Our Sons* (1991), the relationship of gay lovers Donald and James is summarized in words as their being "very close friends," and it is represented in images of the two men playing cards in Donald's hospital room, watching an old Hollywood musical together, and engaging in a bear hug. In *Citizen Cohn* (1992), a sexual relationship between communist headhunter Roy Cohn (played by James Woods) and his male lover is represented by Cohn jumping out of a bed shared with his sleeping lover, having his facial hair shaved and receiving a deathbed hug from the man; and a sexual relationship between the director and deputy director of the FBI is summarized in dialogue explaining that they have been "living together as man and wife" for three decades. In another example, the movie *In the Gloaming* (1997) depicts the entire romantic and sexual relationship between gay son Danny (played by Robert Sean Leonard) and his lover of many years solely through Danny's affirmative responses to his mother's questions as to whether or not he has ever truly loved and whether he was loved in return. Finally, in *One Night Stand* (1997), heterosexual sexual activity is graphically presented in several scenes, but intimacy between gay men is limited to a brief glimpse of Charlie's (played by Robert Downey Jr.) male lover lying in a hospital bed with him during a group visit by Charlie's large circle of friends.

Despite the increased number of gay characters represented on American movie theater and television screens, the recent uproar surrounding comments by the producer of the 1996 AIDS movie

Breaking the Surface: The Greg Louganis Story suggests the amount of representational progress that remains yet unachieved. During a press conference, producer Jim Green was asked to explain why the movie contains scenes of violence between gay male lovers but not two men kissing. Green responded that the audience would be unwilling to watch the latter type of content, and that if audience members tuned out, they would miss the message the movie was designed to send (*GLAAD Images*, 1997, p. 4). Green feared that realistic representations of intimacy between gay men in this movie would detract from the goal of creating "a general awareness and hopefully tolerance for those who are different" (Green/Epstein Productions, 1997). His comments suggest that tolerance of homosexuality in American society can be achieved only at the cost of concealing realities central to being homosexual. The final edit of this movie contains a brutal rape scene of one gay man by another, but no realistic representation of gay male sexual intimacy. The result was an outpouring of criticism from gay activist groups and members of both the gay and mainstream press.

Considering the degree to which heterosexual sexual activity is graphically represented in American movies, such repressive representations of gay male sexuality in AIDS movies targeted to mainstream audiences readily reinforce the pervasive influence of heterosexism as a powerful ideological force in American life. In addition, they do little to alter or expand the typical ways in which nongays perceive gay males and their lived realities.

The preceding discussion is not intended to suggest that no positive representations of gay men in AIDS movies defy the trends just presented. The AIDS movies *Philadelphia* (1993) and *Jeffrey* (1995), for example, are noteworthy for their representations of positive relationships between gay men and both of their parents. The AIDS movies *Men in Love* (1989), *Our Sons* (1991), and *Love! Valour! Compassion!* (1997) are noteworthy for their positive representations of gay lovers in committed, monogamous relationships. Many of the smaller number of AIDS movies that have been created under the guidance of gay directors and/or targeted largely to gay male viewers in the form of independent theatrical releases—including *Jerker* (1991), *The Living End* (1992), *Grief* (1993), *World and Time Enough* (1995), and *Chocolate Babies* (1996)—are notewor-

thy for their more daring and uninhibited representations of gay
male intimacy and sexual activity.

Nevertheless, as explained in Chapter 1, concerns regarding the
social effects of media representations focus primarily on representational trends and the cumulative messages communicated by a
range of related representations rather than on the messages communicated by individual, isolated representations. In this regard,
although the regular representation of gay men in AIDS movies
offered the potential to alter and expand the commonly accepted
ways in which nongays perceive and discuss the status of gay men
and their lived realities in American society, the resulting representations have not lived up to this potential. Even the most typical
positive representation of gay men in AIDS movies—as devoted,
supportive, caretaking, nurturing companions to friends and lovers
dying of AIDS—some researchers fear, perpetuates stereotypes of
gay men by linking them with the traditional nurturing role of
women, thereby reinforcing perceptions of gay men as deviant because they are not really "men" (Pilipp and Shull, 1993, p. 25).

Media representations matter because they are a form of social
action, involving the production of meanings that ultimately have
real effects. As film scholar Richard Dyer explains, the way that
social groups are treated in media representations is frequently part
and parcel of the way they are treated in real life—poverty, harassment, self-hatred, discrimination, and other undesirable outcomes
are instituted and solidified by representation (1993, p. 1). Since AIDS
entered the American consciousness in the early 1980s, gay men have
encountered renewed waves of prejudice and intolerance in American
society. After a generation of growing social tolerance for homosexuality, the persistent representational link between gay men and AIDS has
contributed to the generation of a new homophobia, which has resulted
in harassment and violence toward gay men that is connected to AIDS-
related fears and prejudices (Croteau and Morgan, 1989, p. 86). Formal
"hate campaigns" launched against gay men claim that the AIDS
pandemic is reasonable "evidence" of why their deviance must be
eradicated (Ibid.), and gay men have been physically brutalized by
others who believe them to be the cause of the pandemic (Rushing,
1995, p. 5). In New York City alone, for instance, attacks against gay
men increased from 176 in 1984 to 517 in 1987, with authorities there

attributing most of the increase to the perception of AIDS as a gay disease (Zuckerman, 1988, p. 24). In addition, because representations of AIDS in mass media offerings have so persistently been linked with gay men, many people have attempted to isolate themselves from AIDS by avoiding contact with gay men (Rushing, 1995, p. 159; Sobnosky and Hauser, 1999, p. 31).

The degree to which negative representations of gay men in AIDS movies have influenced negative treatment of gay men in American society during the first two decades of the AIDS pandemic will never be known; however, there is simply no denying that, overall, the makers of these movies passed up significant opportunities to disseminate more positive and realistic representations of gay men and their lived realities to nongay viewers nationwide. The resulting state of affairs is all the more disappointing in light of preliminary experimental research findings revealing that exposure to positive media representations of gay men can have significant positive effects on audience member attitudes, resulting in reduced levels of prejudice toward gay men (Riggle, Ellis, and Crawford, 1996, p. 64).

By associating gay men so persistently with AIDS, while not significantly enhancing representations of gay men and the gay male experience, the regular representation of gay men in AIDS movies has served primarily to reinforce the social construction of AIDS as "a universal problem perpetuated by gays" (Netzhammer and Shamp, 1994, p. 92). As communication scholars Emile Netzhammer and Scott Shamp have noted, this continuous association of homosexuality with AIDS, that is the widely shared perception of AIDS as a "gay disease," can be extremely detrimental, given the changing demographics of the AIDS pandemic (Ibid., p. 103). "As the spread of AIDS in the gay community decreases and transmission in other sectors of the population increases," they explain, "the validity of such a view is growing tenuous" (Ibid.).

CONSEQUENCES OF THE PERSISTENT REPRESENTATIONAL LINK BETWEEN GAY MEN AND AIDS FOR MEMBERS OF OTHER SOCIAL GROUPS

Movies about AIDS, similar to other narrative media offerings, are believed to offer unique possibilities for educating all kinds of viewers about HIV/AIDS and influencing their preventive beha-viors. In part, this is because entertainment offerings containing pertinent information about social issues benefit from a variety of appealing elements of popular culture, including the following:

1. Pervasiveness: entertainment offerings are available every-where.
2. Popularity: most viewers enjoy being entertained.
3. Personal focus: viewers of these offerings are typically moved to share the experience of their characters.
4. Persuasiveness: the messages and characters in these offerings can sway audience members in various ways.
5. Passion: the messages in these offerings can stir strong audience emotions and reactions. (Svenkerud, Rao, and Rogers, 1999, p. 244)

In addition, such offerings include audience members as partici-pants rather than simply as targets, and they can be instrumental in encouraging discussion and debate about the social issues and infor-mation they contain, under certain conditions (Svenkerud, Rao, and Rogers, 1999, p. 244). One such condition involves the homophily of characters in such offerings with viewers, defined as the degree to which the characters are similar to the viewers (Rogers and Shefner-Rogers, 1999, p. 412). The greater the homophily between the central characters in a narrative work and the individual viewing the work, the greater the chance that the work will be considered credible by that viewer, and the greater the chance that the viewer will be influenced personally by it (Ibid.).

Clearly, the persistent representational link between gay men and AIDS in AIDS movies and related media offerings has deflected attention away from the realities of the worldwide pandemic, in which AIDS is overwhelmingly the result of heterosexual sexual transmission (Herek and Glunt, 1988, p. 888). As a result, although HIV/AIDS can be transmitted readily through heterosexual inter-course, many heterosexual Americans have come to view them-selves as inherently different from gay men, thus creating a psycho-logical boundary that makes them feel "protected" from the pandemic (Clark, 1999, p. 9). As AIDS researcher Kevin Clark has noted, heterosexuals have come to believe themselves safe from the pandemic by their self-identification as nongay. He explains that because gay men typically are not visibly distinguishable from straight men, it became desirable for heterosexuals, during the early years of the AIDS pandemic, to devise some sort of classification scheme that could more reliably differentiate one group from the other, and that codified heterosexual behavior as normal and gay male behavior as abnormal (Ibid., p. 13). The resulting conflation of high-risk groups with high-risk behaviors, as Clark points out, thus "rhetorically maintains boundaries between gay and straight communities and so the cultural perception that straights are not at risk for HIV transmission, regardless of their behavior, as long as they stay within the culturally straight community" (Ibid.).

The social construction of the AIDS pandemic as one in which HIV is spread primarily through male-to-male sex, therefore, has sent quite a dangerous message to heterosexual Americans, many of whom probably believe that they are "more likely to be struck by a personal lightning bolt from God" than to become infected with HIV/AIDS (Slagle, 1999, p. 102). In other words, the social construction and representational reinforcement of AIDS as a gay disease reduces its salience for the millions of other Americans who are also at risk and inhibits preventive behaviors (Netzhammer and Shamp, 1994, p. 103).

Although HIV/AIDS continues to spread through the gay community today, its incidence among gay men has remained relatively steady in recent years (*Between the Lines,* 1999, p. 18). In contrast, the transmission of HIV/AIDS through the heterosexual community has been increasing in recent years at alarming rates. Statistics provided by the CDC, for example, reveal that heterosexual women, heterosexual adolescents, and heterosexual African-American men now make up sizable high-risk groups for HIV transmission and AIDS (Wright, 1997, pp. 77-79). It is unfortunate, then, that, at a time when AIDS has become a leading cause of death among twenty-five- to forty-four-year-old Americans of various sexual orientations, most AIDS movies still typically represent the person with AIDS as a gay white male (*Out Post,* 1998, p. 11), and that the few AIDS movies featuring central characters who are members of the heterosexual high-risk groups previously identified have all contained noteworthy shortcomings.

Heterosexual white women who acquired HIV/AIDS through heterosexual sexual activity have been represented as central characters in only two of the AIDS movies analyzed in this study, *Boys on the Side* (1994) and *A Mother's Prayer* (1995); heterosexual women of color who acquired HIV/AIDS in the same way have virtually been ignored. *Boys on the Side* stands out as one of the only AIDS movies that has apparently attempted intentionally to avoid the persistent representational link between gay men and AIDS entirely: it features a central female character with AIDS as its only AIDS character, and it does not represent nor refer to gay men in any way.

In *Boys on the Side,* Robin (played by Mary-Louise Parker) contracted HIV from a heterosexual male bartender, and her HIV status is treated in this movie as just another part of her sexual history. For reasons that are unclear, however, *Boys on the Side* fails to make a clean break from associating AIDS with homosexuality in some way. Robin's close companion in the movie is Jane (played by Whoopi Goldberg), a lesbian performer who is secretly in love with her straight friend and who is constantly referred to by their mutual friend Holly (played by Drew Barrymore) as being "gay." Thus, while representing the person with AIDS as an individual who falls outside the socially constructed, ideological risk group category of gay men, this AIDS movie, nevertheless, includes elements that repeatedly bring homosexuality and "gayness" to mind. The work has also been criticized for the decision to portray a white woman with AIDS and her black sidekick rather than portraying a black woman with AIDS and her white sidekick. This criticism came about because, at the time the movie was released, statistics provided by the CDC revealed that one out of five deaths among black women in the United States, ages twenty-five to forty-four, was caused by AIDS, a reality the movie entirely ignores (Hogan, 1998, p. 170).

Similarly, although *A Mother's Prayer* focuses on the efforts of a heterosexual woman named Rosemary (played by Linda Hamilton), to find a new home for her son before she succumbs to AIDS (she became infected through sex with her husband), the persistent link between gay men and AIDS is inadvertently reinforced in the movie by the inclusion of actor/singer RuPaul, starring as a gay man with

AIDS who befriends the dying woman, and by the reality that several key scenes play out at the Gay Men's Health Crisis offices in New York City. Of the seventy-six AIDS characters in the thirty-two AIDS movies analyzed, only 14.5 percent (n = 11) are female, whereas 85.5 percent (n = 65) are male.

Heterosexual adolescents who acquired HIV/AIDS through heterosexual sexual transmission have been represented as central characters in just two of the other AIDS movies analyzed in this study, *Something to Live For: The Alison Gertz Story* (1992) and *Kids* (1995). Although *Something to Live For* recounts the real-life story of Alison Gertz, who contracted HIV at age sixteen during a one-night stand with a bartender at Studio 54 and died of AIDS a decade later, its most noteworthy shortcoming is that it is targeted primarily to an older television-movie-of-the-week crowd rather than to adolescents themselves. As such, it is a bit too conservative in its narrative, dialogue, and visuals to appeal to many of today's teens, and the homophily between Alison—an affluent young woman from a good family on New York's Upper East Side who enjoys quite a conservative lifestyle—and the majority of modern teens is lacking.

In contrast, *Kids* goes to the opposite extreme in attempting to appeal to today's adolescents by including unrestrained profanity ("fuck," "shit," and "pussy," for example, are all spoken in the opening sequence, followed immediately by "motherfucking"); images of public urination, shoplifting, endless partying, extreme violence, and two young women kissing; graphic sex scenes and lengthy graphic discussions about "fucking" and "sucking dick"; and a powerful rock and heavy metal soundtrack. AIDS activists maintain that graphic representations such as these can be far more effective than less explicit, clinical depictions at reaching adolescents and getting them to reflect on health risks stemming from their own sexual practices (McCoy, Miles, and Metsch, 1999, p. 43; Nelson, 1999, p. 57). In addition, the homophily between the movie's central characters and many modern teens is a bit improved here. The primary shortcoming of this AIDS movie, however, is that the extremely wild and uncontrolled lifestyle of all of the adolescents represented in it may lead many more responsible teens to

believe that their own, more restrained personal behavior will ultimately protect them from the health risks presented.

Another shortcoming of both of these AIDS movies is their inclusion of gay male characters as part of their narratives. In *Something to Live For,* Alison's gay friend, Peter, appears sporadically to
point out that half of his friends are now dead from AIDS and that,
despite his own HIV-negative health status and responsible sexual
behavior, he is nevertheless concerned about getting AIDS every
minute of every day, which suggests that contracting AIDS is an
almost inevitable outcome for gay men in modern American society, even when they are limiting their number of sexual partners and
consistently engaging in safer sexual practices. In *Kids,* a park
scene following Jennie's (played by Chloe Sevigny) discovery that
she has been infected with HIV by Telly (played by Leo Fitzpatrick)
unnecessarily features two butch gay men walking hand in hand and
several of the male teens calling them "sick" and "fucking faggots."
By focusing on heterosexual sexual transmission of AIDS, these
two movies have the potential to undermine the perception of AIDS
as a "gay disease" by incorporating characters who contract HIV/
AIDS by nongay means. In the end, however, they fail to live up to
that potential by ultimately being unable to resist the persistent
temptation to introduce gay characters and homosexuality into every
story about AIDS (Netzhammer and Shamp, 1994, p. 103). Accordingly, these two movies, similar to the ones mentioned in the discussion of heterosexual women, ultimately maintain the link between
AIDS and gay male sexuality. Of the seventy-six AIDS characters in
the thirty-two AIDS movies analyzed, only 7.9 percent (n = 6) are
teenagers, whereas 92.1 percent (n = 70) are adults.

Finally, heterosexual African-American men who acquired HIV/
AIDS through heterosexual sexual activity have yet to be represented
as central characters in any of the AIDS movies analyzed in this study.
Of the seventy-six AIDS characters in the thirty-two AIDS movies
analyzed, only six (7.9 percent) are African American, five of whom
are gay males and one of whom is a heterosexual female. It is perhaps
also noteworthy that four of these six characters appear in the same
AIDS movie, *Chocolate Babies* (1996). For comparison's sake, with
regard to race and ethnicity, 84.2 percent (n = 64) of the AIDS characters in these movies are white, 5.3 percent (n = 4) are Hispanic, and

2.6 percent (n = 2) fall into the category of "other" (one is Israeli, and the other is half Samoan). It is possible that the apparent reluctance to represent minorities as people with AIDS in AIDS movies extends from concerns that doing so might fuel stereotypes about members of minority groups or increase racial tensions (Goldstein, 1991, p. 27). The end result, however, has served to deprive such individuals of essential information they need regarding the actual extent of their HIV/AIDS risk (Ibid.).

As long as individuals in specific demographic groups continue to believe that members of their group are not significantly at risk for HIV/AIDS transmission, they are far less likely to engage in safer sexual practices themselves than if they more accurately perceived the realistic health risks they and other members of their group face. AIDS in American society is no longer a disease of "the other" when viewed from the vantage point of most sexually active individuals, whether or not those individuals actually understand this to be the case. More regular representations of AIDS that convey the wide range of Americans at risk for contracting and transmitting HIV/AIDS hold the potential to more fully inform various (nongay) individuals of their own health risks, so that they may begin taking the pandemic more seriously and reconsider whether they need to modify their current sexual practices in favor of more consistently engaging in safer sexual practices.

In the United States today, women make up the fastest-growing group of people with HIV/AIDS (Stevens and Bogart, 1999, p. 107); the HIV infection rate of women is increasing at four times the rate of men (Roth and Fuller, 1998, p. 1). Recent findings of a survey conducted jointly by Yale University and Music Television (MTV) reveal that nearly nine out of ten young people living in the United States today do not feel that they are vulnerable to contracting the AIDS retrovirus, even though 20 percent of the respondents indicated that they knew of someone who had already died of AIDS (*Between the Lines,* 1999, p. 17). Although African Americans represent only 13 percent of our nation's population, they account for nearly half of all new AIDS cases reported today; similarly, although Hispanics represent only 10 percent of America's population, they account for more than 20 percent of new AIDS cases (Zupan, 1998, p. 13). So why is it that the persistent representational link between gay men and AIDS has been reinforced so significantly, even in five of the six most recent AIDS movies analyzed in this study, to the detriment of gay males as well as members of various other social groups?

The social construction of AIDS as a gay disease, in conjunction with the culturally shared distancing formula that produces the perception that AIDS happens to somebody else, inaccurately prevents many Americans from considering themselves to be at risk for HIV/AIDS (Estrada and Quintero, 1999, p. 135). The resulting state of affairs is quite disconcerting because, although it is presently noncurable, HIV/AIDS is almost always preventable (Ibid., p. 134). Although understanding AIDS as a gay disease has been "easy" and "comfortable" for the majority of Americans to date, the time is long overdue for AIDS movies and related mass media offerings to break the long-standing, largely counterproductive connection between gay men and AIDS and more fully explore alternate ways of "humanizing" the pandemic (Netzhammer and Shamp, 1994, pp. 105-106). As so many AIDS activists have argued, it is only when the public at large truly appreciates the impact of HIV/AIDS on all of American society that we can seriously begin to address the AIDS crisis (Sobnosky and Hauser, 1999, p. 28).

Chapter 5

AIDS and the City
(versus the Country)

"The role played by the city is central to a wide variety of films," explains David Clarke, in his preface to the anthology *The Cinematic City*, "[y]et the relationship between city and cinema has been neglected in both film and urban studies" (1997, p. i). As Clarke observes, the representation of cities in movies has occurred from cinema's earliest days to the present, with perceptions of cities (in opposition to rural settings) being unmistakably molded by the resulting representations (Ibid., p. 1). For this reason, he finds it surprising that scholars, to date, have not yet devoted adequate attention to exploring the seemingly complex connections between movies and cities. "So central is the city to [movies]," Clarke notes, "that, paradoxically, the widespread implicit acceptance of its importance has mitigated against an explicit consideration of its actual significance" (Ibid.).

The present chapter provides an exploration of the representational connections between the city (versus the country) and the AIDS movie. Traditionally, representations of cities in movies have focused variously on the attractive and repulsive qualities of the city, which have derived historically from various social and moral oppositions associated with the city versus the country: metropolis/small town, words/deeds, hypocrisy/honesty, cash relations/human relations, individual/community, excess/modesty (Mahoney, 1997, p. 178; McArthur, 1997, p. 23). Representations of cities in AIDS movies provide no exception to this trend. In general, two competing representations of the city are provided: the city as gay utopia and the city as AIDS dystopia. Both of these representations of the city are simultaneously contrasted with the predominant representation of the country, which can most effectively be described as all that is good and moral in America, a balm to injured minds and bodies (Ibid., p. 24). As such, the representational distinctions between city versus country provide yet another noteworthy form of otherness encountered in AIDS movies, that contributes significantly to the ongoing social construction of the AIDS pandemic in American society.

THE CITY AS GAY UTOPIA AND AIDS DYSTOPIA

Cities are such an essential component of AIDS movies that the narratives of only 15.6 percent (n = 5) of the AIDS movies analyzed in this study (specifically, *Breaking the Surface: The Greg Louganis Story*, *The Cure*, *A Place for Annie*, *The Ryan White Story*, and *World and Time Enough*) are not linked to a major American city in any significant way. Of the remaining 84.4 percent (n = 27) of AIDS movies that incorporate at least one city as an essential component of their narratives, more than three-fourths of them are set in one or more major American cities (such as New York, Los Angeles, and/or San Francisco) that serve as a backdrop for the majority of their narrative developments, and slightly less than one-fourth feature a central character who heads from city to country (and frequently back to city again) for an extended period of time. As film scholar Colin McArthur notes in his analysis of the elusive cinematic city, all discursive spaces common to media offerings have volatile valencies, with the same spaces typically being utilized in various works to signify somewhat incompatible ideological positions (1997, p. 24). It is not entirely surprising, therefore, that the city is simultaneously (and somewhat contradictorily) represented both as (gay) utopia and (AIDS) dystopia within AIDS movies.

Representations of the city as gay utopia in AIDS movies stem from the traditional draw of America's cities as places of gay liberation and bases for the formation of distinctive gay subcultures. This phenomenon is an extension of the networks of gay men that first appeared in European cities during the late fourteenth century and flourished thereafter (Rushing, 1995, p. 20). By the middle of the twentieth century, distinctive gay subcultures with supportive living spaces and gathering places were common in cities across the

United States. In 1949, for example, urban sociologist Ernest Burgess noted that every major American city contains its own separate homosexual world, with its own language, literature, and codes of conduct, which are somewhat incomprehensible to outsiders while offering sympathy and moral support to members (Ibid.).

Such gay subcultures have historically occupied their own physical and social spaces within America's cities, thereby allowing them to remain figuratively sealed off from surrounding neighborhoods and, therefore, largely out of the view of most outsiders (Rushing, 1995, p. 20). As a result, so-called "gay ghettos"—featuring a wide range of social and political institutions and strong, stable gay identities—have emerged in cities nationwide (Padgug and Oppenheimer, 1992, p. 248). These communities provide supportive subcultural domains in the form of gay bars, sex institutions, special political organizations, community centers, social clubs, and the like to their gay male residents and newcomers from other areas. It is here that many gay men first meet others similar to themselves and feel free to express themselves in ways denied them elsewhere in their lives, providing them with a solid sense of identity, "family," and community (Altman, 1982, p. 21).

This positive state of affairs for gay men has been translated into representations of the city in AIDS movies as a gay utopia. Social information about this gay utopia is communicated to viewers in various ways. Most commonly, this information is communicated through the incorporation of positive representations of groups of gay men serving as reliable support systems for one another in happy times as well as sad. Although examples of this variety can be found in almost any AIDS movie, some of the most noteworthy examples occur in the movies *On Common Ground* (1992), *Chocolate Babies* (1996), *Jeffrey* (1995), and *It's My Party* (1996).

In *On Common Ground,* for example, the city of Los Angeles provides home to a welcoming gay bar, The Purple Parrot, that serves as a supportive gathering spot for gay men and lesbians in the years prior to and during the AIDS pandemic. Within the walls of this establishment, gay men of various class and racial/ethnic backgrounds are shown openly kissing and physically admiring one another, as well as slow dancing together. A core group of loyal gay patrons in this movie—along with new ones as the years go

by—flock to this protective space on a regular basis to engage in more
fulfilling social interactions than are possible in most other areas they
encounter, as well as to freely discuss issues of interest and relevance
to their lives. Such issues range in topic from police brutality toward
homosexuals and burgeoning social activism to the latest episodes of
gay public-access talk shows and the prime-time soap opera *Dynasty*.

Similarly, in *Chocolate Babies,* New York City serves both as the
center of AIDS activism and the center of romantic, sexual, and
supportive relationships for a band of gay men (and one straight
woman) who confront conservative politicians about their indiffer-
ence to the negative social and health realities encountered daily in
communities of color. These individuals are regularly described by
the city's media professionals as "bizarre gay terrorists" and "faggots," solidifying their sense of identification with one another.
Although their goal is to make all of New York City's boroughs safe
for gays and people with AIDS, they focus most of their efforts on
attempting to influence community leaders in their own neighborhood, the blocks surrounding the rooftop location favored by their
leader, Max Mo Freak (played by Claude Sloan Jr.). Max and his
friends pass many hours on a couch atop this high-rise building, from
which they watch over the secure, special subcultural space they
have created for themselves. The romantic relationship between Max
and the younger gay activist Sam blossoms in these supportive surroundings, and they and their friends freely share graphic information about preferred sex acts, sexual relationships past and present,
and conceptions of gay love therein, far removed from the disapproving glances and reactions of nongay others.

In *Jeffrey,* the concept of the city as gay utopia is communicated
through the strong bonds of friendship and continuous emotional
support that develop between four disparate gay characters who call
New York City their home: Jeffrey (played by Steven Weber), an
unemployed New York City actor who has sworn off sex; Steve
(played by Michael T. Weiss), a perpetually horny, HIV-positive
bartender; Darius (played by Bryan Batt), a chorus boy in the musical *Cats;* and Sterling (played by Patrick Stewart), the much older
interior designer. The movie's opening shots of Jeffrey having sex
(or at least attempting to) with several other men provide the first
indication that he lives in one of his city's gay ghettos, where gay

male sexual partners are readily available and homosexuality is accepted as the norm. This initial perception is confirmed minutes later in the movie when Jeffrey goes to his local gym and is kissed passionately by Steve, a new member he has just met; the other men working out around them simply look on and smile in approval. The supportive urban space carved out by Jeffrey, his gay friends, and other members of the gay community features queer-friendly retail establishments with gay personnel and numerous public spaces in which it is not considered at all out of the ordinary for gay men to hold hands, hug, kiss, dance together, or bring each other flowers. Life within this gay ghetto, as Darius explains to Jeffrey, is enjoyed as one big party by its residents; scenes from a gay pride parade reveal the diversity of gay residents who coexist peacefully and respectfully therein. Naturally, this special subcultural domain must remain protected from disapproving (straight) outsiders, which explains why Sterling and Darius become members of the Pink Panthers, an organized patrol to prevent gay bashing. Through their participation, they also strengthen their identification as residents of a supportive gay ghetto in which they, and others similar to them, can thrive.

Finally, in *It's My Party*, members of the supportive LA-based gay community enjoyed by Nick (played by Eric Roberts), Brandon (played by Gregory Harrison), and their friends come through for one another consistently, in good times and in bad. Gay doctors provide more caring treatment to their gay patients, gay men in love freely reveal this reality to others through their various words and actions, and older gay men provide advice about life and love to younger ones. The extensive support network enabled by the concentration of gay men in this subcultural city-based domain offers continuous loyalty, friendship, and a larger sense of "family." As an example, the final-farewell bash in this movie is so well attended by Nick's many supportive gay friends that even Nick's homophobic father is moved to reverse his negative feelings about gay men. Acknowledging that he has been ashamed of Nick from the moment he found out his son was gay, the man points out that observing Nick interacting with his caring friends has made him see things differently.

For viewers who may not fully perceive the benefits offered to gay men in these subcultural urban settings simply by viewing such representations of life within them, another way that social information about the city as gay utopia is communicated more directly is in the form of character dialogue. In *It's My Party*, for example, as Nick is preparing to take his own life with pills, his ex-lover, Brandon, explains to members of Nick's circle of friends that the Greeks believed it is not horrible to die but rather to die alone; one of Nick's friends responds that it would be impossible for Nick to do so because in the gay community one gets to choose his family, and Nick chose all of them. In similar fashion, the character Bobbi Campbell (played by Donal Logue) in *And the Band Played On* (1993) explains that because he had always been labeled a "freak" in his conservative hometown as a result of his "deviant" sexual orientation, he was thrilled to arrive in San Francisco where he found a community of others similar to himself. He emphasizes that in the Castro District, gay men stick together and that he would rather die as a human being who is free to have sex with other men, whenever and wherever he desires, than to have continued living his life as a "freak" elsewhere.

Yet another noteworthy example of this process occurs in the 1991 AIDS movie *Jerker*, in which the character Bert (played by Tom Wagner) characterizes the Castro District as being like a new Midwest (since so many gay men relocate there from the actual Midwest) in which individuals considered to be deviant in other areas can successfully live and work, survive and thrive, and have consenting sex with others on as frequent a basis as desired. As an example, he describes one of his friends who died recently of AIDS as a fun, attractive, resourceful, and horny hairstylist who had sex with many of his customers right in his barber's chair.

What is particularly interesting about these and related representations of the city as gay utopia in AIDS movies is how inextricably they are linked, both explicitly and implicitly, to representations of the city as AIDS dystopia. In these latter sorts of representations, the city is presented as a site of transcendental (rather than social) alienation in which human life is experienced, ultimately, as being somewhat unfulfilling because something essential (even if not readily identifiable) is felt to be missing (Easthope, 1997, p. 133).

This something can be determined to be a successful existence without the constant lurking threat of AIDS. As such, the city is represented to be the place of AIDS infection, where death and dying make up a depressingly regular component of everyday life.

As gender studies scholar Cindy Patton has observed about the initial identification of HIV/AIDS by physicians in America's urban areas, the emerging syndrome that ultimately became known as AIDS was initially identified as an immune malfunction in individuals who were previously considered by doctors and researchers to be healthy individuals (1990, p. 28). "That gay men were seen as 'healthy' despite having a variety of treatable sexually transmitted diseases attested to the acceptance and positive valuation of gay men and their sexuality in the urban settings where these early cases were under study," Patton explains. "Had these cases appeared fifty years ago, and had the homosexuality of the patients been recognized, doctors would probably have viewed homosexuals *per se* as constitutionally weaker and explained their immune system breakdown on this fact alone" (Ibid). In other words, the success of the American city as gay utopia is terminologically evident in the way in which physicians have discussed HIV/AIDS from the pandemic's earliest days. At the same time, however, it is this same success that is considered to be largely responsible for the rapid spread of AIDS throughout the gay community from its earliest days.

As sociologist William Rushing has noted, a social paradox of successful gay liberation is that it produced changes in gay male sexual activity that were destined to become important factors in the AIDS pandemic (1995, p. 24). He explains that as gay sexual freedom increased in America's cities, the number of sex institutions (such as bathhouses, bars with dark "fuck rooms" in the back, porn theaters, massage parlors, and "tearooms") increased as well to meet the needs of sexual desire, helping to produce sex-positive norms of polygamous gay sex that ultimately guaranteed the rapid spread of HIV/AIDS through the gay population, and eventually to members of various other social groups (Ibid., pp. 24-25, 32).

An estimate of how quickly the pandemic spread through cities with strong gay subcultures is suggested by the percentage of gay men visiting the same San Francisco-based sexually transmitted disease (STD) clinic who tested positive for HIV: 1 percent in 1978,

25 percent in 1980, and 65 percent in 1984 (Rushing, 1995, p. 32). By the mid-1980s, many Americans hoped that AIDS would stay within its "natural limits" of urban gay communities (Clark, 1999, p. 13), a view that has unmistakably influenced representations of the city in AIDS movies as an AIDS dystopia. Journalists at that time typically constructed their stories and images of people with AIDS in such a way as to emphasize the otherness of members of this group, relying heavily on urban locations and their inhabitants as a form of representational shorthand for signifying the "anonymous, potentially dangerous urban gay man" (Cook and Colby, 1992, p. 95).

As with representations of the city as gay utopia, social information about the city as AIDS dystopia is communicated to viewers of AIDS movies in various ways. Occasionally, it is communicated implicitly by powerful images of the city, such as in the 1992 AIDS movie *Chain of Desire,* which presents a daisy chain of sexual encounters between members of the same trendy Manhattan set. In the end, after the "patient zero" in this chain reveals that he is HIV positive and urges the second sexual participant to get tested, the film concludes with powerful night images of New York City shot from above, calling to mind the potential number of city residents who may be engaging in similar sexual encounters and transmitting HIV/AIDS at that moment. In a related way, images of urban life from cities such as New York and San Francisco appear regularly throughout the 1990 AIDS movie *Longtime Companion,* making it clear to the viewer that all of the gay central characters shown suffering and/or dying from AIDS in this offering are devoted city dwellers. From start to finish, this movie represents the city as an especially depressing place to live because so many gay men there keep losing so many of their loved ones to AIDS. In contrast to such representation of the city, *Longtime Companion* also represents the countryside and beach communities as places where gay men can escape the stresses associated with urban life and the far greater chances of contracting HIV/AIDS in the city.

More frequently, social information about the city as AIDS dystopia is communicated explicitly to viewers in the form of character dialogue, such as when the character James (played by Hugh Grant) in the 1991 AIDS movie *Our Sons* mentions that he and his gay lover have been to more than a dozen funerals in the past year and a half, or when the character Dean (played by Eric Swanson) in the 1994 AIDS movie *Under Heat* is asked about his friends in the city and responds that, although he has made several friends there, most of them are now dead. In similar fashion, in the 1989 AIDS movie *Men in Love*, the character Steven (played by Doug Self) harshly criticizes a gay acquaintance, Robert (played by Emerald Starr), for living peacefully in a Hawaiian paradise while simultaneously turning his back entirely on their mutual friends with AIDS on the mainland. As he does so, Steven emphasizes the quantities of diarrhea and vomit that he has been forced to clean up day after day while caring for various city-dwelling friends and loved ones with AIDS. He also explains how painful it is to witness so many individuals suffering from dementia in the final stages of their battles with the disease, as well as the extreme pain he feels when his friends ultimately lose those battles.

A popular variation on this direct approach involves city-dwelling characters in AIDS movies who frequently verbalize their desire to get out of the city before it gets them. For example, the HIV-positive character Nick (played by Steve Buscemi) in the 1986 AIDS movie *Parting Glances* informs an uninfected gay friend that his male lover has the right idea about leaving New York City and that he should get out, too, suggesting that the man head for somewhere such as Wisconsin, Colorado, or Virginia. In another example, the title character in the 1995 AIDS movie *Jeffrey* announces that he is leaving New York City for Wisconsin, where he hopes to hide out until the entire AIDS pandemic is over. Similarly, the central AIDS character, Robin (played by Mary-Louise Parker), in the 1994 AIDS movie *Boys on the Side* departs New York City for points West because she believes that if she simply goes somewhere else she can make her own experience confronting HIV/AIDS not happen.

A third way that social information about the city as AIDS dystopia is communicated to viewers is through the story lines of various AIDS movies. In *Breaking the Surface: The Greg Louganis Story* (1996), Tom's illicit gay activities in the city of Los Angeles (including his stint as a male prostitute) condemn both himself and his lover to infection with HIV/AIDS; and in *Gia* (1998), the title character's newfound trendy lifestyle in New York City lures her into experimenting with the readily available intravenous drugs that result in her contracting and dying from HIV/AIDS. Similarly, the plot of *Something to Live For: The Alison Gertz Story* (1992) strongly suggests that AIDS runs so rampant in the city that just one instance of unprotected sex, typically, will kill, as does the plot of *Kids* (1995), which represents the dystopian city as the place where AIDS spreads wildly and uncontrollably to Americans of all ages.

Clearly, AIDS movies consistently take "real" American cities such as New York, Los Angeles, and San Francisco and reinscribe them into discourse once again, transforming them into powerful signifiers of particular ideologies that contribute to the social construction of HIV/AIDS (McArthur, 1997, p. 33). Although on the surface the representation of the city as gay utopia appears to be far more positive in its ideological valence than the representation of the city as AIDS dystopia, the distinction between the two becomes quite blurred when contrasted with the predominant representation of the country as all that is good and moral in American society. That is because representations of the city as either gay utopia or AIDS dystopia, nevertheless, always stem from conditions identifiable in their real-world counterparts, which contain significant doses of "deviance"—with regard to sexual orientation, sexual freedom, sexual promiscuity, and/or sexually transmitted health conditions—as it is socially defined, and which the country (as a representational ideal) presumably never encounters.

THE COUNTRY AS BALM
TO CITY-DWELLING "DEVIANTS"

For many decades, the hegemonic ideologies of American life have valorized the country over the city (McArthur, 1997, p. 32). Within the domain of cinematic history, the country has traditionally signified all that is considered to be good and moral in American society, in striking contrast to the evil temptations that lurk around every corner in the city. Within the domain of AIDS movies, more specifically, the inherent goodness of the country and its residents is continually contrasted with the immorality of the city and of the "deviants" who dwell there. The effective communication of this ideological contrast is ensured through the regular construction of

AIDS movie narratives that feature such city dwellers seeking refuge from the city in the country by traveling from one to the other (and sometimes back again), with the rural environs they temporarily inhabit serving as a balm to their injured minds and/or bodies (Ibid., p. 24).

The AIDS pandemic in the United States has predominantly been socially constructed as a phenomenon that is alien to the country's natural order of things, even though people with HIV/AIDS certainly live throughout rural America. As previously mentioned, this construction results in large part from media accounts framing AIDS and people with AIDS as primarily an urban (rather than rural) health threat. An outstanding example of this process is offered by the NBC news report from May 6, 1985, about a rural hemophiliac who passed HIV/AIDS along to his wife and young child, in which the anchor referred to the family's unfortunate situation as an extreme tragedy far surpassing the number of individuals involved because those individuals lived in a mobile home in central Pennsylvania, far away from gay enclaves in New York City or San Francisco (Cook and Colby, 1992, p. 96). Stories such as this one readily foster the perception that people with HIV/AIDS do not exist nor belong in the country, where their otherness threatens all that is (and those who are) represented to be moral and good. Accordingly, it becomes a bit clearer, ideologically, as to why AIDS characters who seek refuge or even redemption in the country (or at least in more rural settings) are not allowed to remain there indefinitely—they must either return to the city to be with "their own kind" or die a ready death.

In the 1992 AIDS movie *Chain of Desire,* New York City resident Michael, upon learning that he is HIV positive, announces that he is leaving the big city and heading back to his childhood home. His statement indicates that he will not ultimately remain there but, rather, will eventually return to the city. Apparently, Michael senses the lesson learned by other AIDS characters in AIDS movies such as *An Early Frost* (1985), *Philadelphia* (1993), *Under Heat* (1994), and *Love! Valour! Compassion!* (1997): the country is a nice place to visit, but you will not be allowed to live there (permanently).

In *An Early Frost,* for example, Michael (played by Aidan Quinn) returns to the country from Chicago and reveals to his family members that he is gay and has AIDS. He wrestles with their diverse reactions, that he, as the "contaminated stranger," is expected to leave his biological family and return to his "own kind" in the big city, the place of gay men and AIDS (Pilipp and Schull, 1993, p. 22). Michael has no idea what awaits him in his struggle with AIDS, but he knows that he wants to face the challenges ahead with support from his lover, Peter (played by D. W. Moffett), and Michael's father has made it clear that neither his son nor his son's lover are especially welcome outside of the city. When Michael begs his father (played by Ben Gazzara) to reconsider his disapproving reactions toward him, the man replies that Michael cannot return home unexpectedly on his own terms and expect others to react the way he wants them to; things outside the city do not work that way. The father refers to his son as a "stranger," an unknown other who has become so only since he became corrupted by the immoral lures of the city. As such, the situation only worsens when Peter visits Michael at his parents' rural home. The father remains cold and distant in all of his (superficial) interactions with his son's lover, and he makes it perfectly clear how unwelcome Peter is in this rural environment by indicating that he wishes Peter had contracted HIV/AIDS rather than Michael. The message to both son and lover is communicated loudly and clearly. Peter returns immediately to the couple's gay ghetto in Chicago; Michael follows just days later, with his parents making no mention of their door being open to him should he need any assistance during his battle with AIDS.

Similar sentiments are communicated through the narratives of other AIDS movies with regard to AIDS characters who venture out of the city and into more rural settings. In *Philadelphia,* although his most supportive family moments occur at his parents' rural home rather than in the city, Andrew Beckett (played by Tom Hanks) is nevertheless destined to die in the cold, sterile surroundings of an urban hospital rather than in the warmth of a loving home environment, with his relatives simply dropping by to say goodbye. In *Under Heat,* HIV-positive Dean (played by Eric Swanson) visits the country to inform his mother and brother of his compromised health condition. With that deed done, he falls in love and has sex with a younger HIV-positive man; thereafter, he and his new gay lover must return immediately to the city because, as Dean's older brother reminds him, they have laws against such immoral activities in the country. In *Love! Valour! Compassion!*, the HIV-positive gay men Buzz and James (played by Jason Alexander and John Glover, respectively) find love at the country home of a friend on summer holidays, yet (seemingly) because they are the only two gay men who visit there regularly who also have AIDS, they are never invited to remain there for extended periods. After an occasional day or two of relief from the grind of city life, they are banished from the comforting balm of the country and forced by their various ties and commitments to return to different cities thereafter, where they eventually die outside of each other's arms.

AIDS characters who opt instead to remain in a country setting to partake of its balm to their injured minds and bodies on an extended basis, rather than returning to the city in a timely fashion, apparently must be eradicated through an even more rapid death to protect the country's pure and moral nature from the ongoing negative influence of these "deviant" and "contaminated" strangers. Consider, for example, the experiences of Robin (played by Mary-Louise Parker) in the 1994 AIDS movie *Boys on the Side*. After fleeing New York City in an attempt to restore her health in a more wholesome setting, Robin finds that she begins to thrive in the desert home she shares with two friends. Her T-cell count increases dramatically, and her body no longer shows any outward signs of illness. The situation goes downhill quickly, however, after Robin meets the straight rural bartender Alex (played by James Remar), who wants to have sex with her. Although Alex does not seem to attach much significance to Robin's HIV-positive status and seeks virtually to overlook it because he is so horny, Robin points out that Alex can no longer simply get drunk, have a wild time, and engage in casual sexual encounters because AIDS has spread outside the boundaries of the city and the infected Robin has settled in to stay. Minutes later in the movie, Robin suffers a serious health setback; soon afterward, she withers away and dies. As such, the imminent AIDS threat she posed has been eradicated, restoring (at least for a while) the "purity" of the country from the ongoing negative influence of the deviant and contaminated stranger from New York City.

Similar circumstances are encountered by Danny (played by Robert Sean Leonard) in the 1997 AIDS movie *In the Gloaming,* after he gives up his life in San Francisco and returns to live indefinitely in his parents' country home. Danny's father (played by David Strathairn) makes it immediately clear that he does not welcome his son's continued presence, and his mother (played by Glenn Close) realizes how painful it has been for her son to never be invited home with his gay lover to visit. Here again, it becomes representationally clear that deviant city dwellers—this time in the form of gay men (and especially those with AIDS)—are never truly welcome in the country, where they pose a threat to its more moral social order. As such, it is far from surprising that Danny passes away just several weeks after he arrives, or that his father is interested in getting to know what his son was like only after Danny dies, and, therefore, can no longer pose any real threat to the "purity" of the country.

Certainly, the regular representation of the city as gay utopia/ AIDS dystopia in AIDS movies—in opposition to (as well as in conjunction with) the representation of the country as the good, pure, moral balm to city-dwelling deviants—dangerously reinforces outdated culturally shared notions of HIV/AIDS as a plague of the city and a threatening phenomenon of concern almost exclusively to residents there. The pervasive nature of these predominant representations of urban and nonurban geographical spaces serves to conceal much needed, accurate social information about the "true nature" of AIDS in the increasingly geographically boundless modern age.

Chapter 6

Other Ways of Representing AIDS

Not all representations of AIDS in American movies occur in narrative "AIDS movies," as defined in Chapter 1 of this work and explored in the preceding five chapters. At times, AIDS characters are introduced into non-AIDS movies in ways that are incidental to their narratives, or characters with symptoms similar to those of HIV/AIDS are featured in movies that do not directly represent AIDS, yet do so metaphorically. At other times, individuals living with (and dying from) AIDS opt to represent themselves in documentaries made with the assistance of trusted associates and friends, in an attempt to save the lives of viewers by more realistically depicting conditions encountered by people in the final stages of AIDS, thereby reemphasizing the importance of consistently protecting oneself from the threat of the pandemic to as great an extent as possible.

The present chapter focuses on these various alternative approaches to representing AIDS. It begins with an exploration of the form and function of AIDS characters in non-AIDS movies, and it proceeds to discussions of AIDS metaphor movies and self-representation in AIDS documentaries. The chapter concludes with an update on the current status of HIV/AIDS transmission in American society and the corresponding need for representing AIDS in unique ways during the third decade of AIDS and (likely) beyond.

THE FORM AND FUNCTION
OF AIDS CHARACTERS IN NON-AIDS MOVIES

The first alternative approach to representing AIDS in movies involves the inclusion of AIDS characters in non-AIDS movies. To date, this approach has been utilized in only a small number of movies, such as *Joey Breaker* (1993), *Second Best* (1994), and *Forrest Gump* (1994). Nevertheless, it is a promising approach that tends to avoid some of the most typical representational shortcomings common to many AIDS movies, as discussed in the preceding five chapters.

The phrase *non-AIDS movie* in this discussion refers specifically to any movie that includes at least one character with HIV/AIDS yet does so in a way that is incidental to its narrative; in other words, the movie could delete all references to HIV/AIDS and achieve similar narrative ends using different narrative means, without significantly altering its plot.

One such movie is *Joey Breaker,* in which Fred Fondren plays Alfred, a former librarian with AIDS who is brought meals occasionally by two employees from the same creative artists agency in Manhattan. One of these employees is agent and title character Joey Breaker (played by Richard Edson), who lives solely for his work and thrives on the rush derived from making a profitable deal. When Joey first accompanies one of his female associates to deliver food to Alfred, he is visibly uncomfortable during the entire encounter, and he reprimands his friend for kissing Alfred good-bye. Disappointed by Joey's reaction, his friend informs Joey that, although he may be a great agent, he is certainly lacking in the life department. The narrative thus becomes one centered on Joey's search to find his true self and deepen his interactions with others. His quest leads him to interact more fully with Alfred, one on one in a few brief scenes; in the process, he discovers that Alfred shares his own passion for the cinema and the two become friends. During a touching scene in which Joey feeds Alfred his food in bed, Alfred reveals that he is not scared to die but that he is angry because, at age forty-six, he regrets all of the things he has not yet done. Days later, Alfred is dead, but his words change Joey's life. Joey begins to treat the clients he represents as individuals rather than as undifferentiated moneymakers, and he starts to explore the meaning of his life outside the professional domain. Ultimately, Joey quits the job he thought he loved to pursue a relationship with Cyan (played by Cedella Marley), a Jamaican waitress and student who has returned to Jamaica to work as a nurse. The movie concludes six months later in their lives, when the couple is living blissfully in a simpler, more fulfilling environment.

Another such movie is *Second Best,* in which Keith Allen plays John, the biological father of a young boy, James (played by Chris Cleary Miles), who is about to be adopted by another man. The other man is Graham Holt (played by William Hurt), a forty-two-year-old postmaster who has had a lifelong strained relationship with his own father and desires to provide an emotionally support-ive environment for the emotionally disturbed youth. For much of his life, James has been shuttled from one children's home to the next as John has served numerous prison sentences. After John relinquishes his parental rights and gives his blessing to the adop-tion, he shows up unexpectedly at the post office, wanting to see the boy. John reveals that he has been released from prison early to spare officials there the need to write one additional death certifi-cate because he is dying of AIDS and does not have long to live. Graham offers to let the man move in and spend the last few months of his life getting to know James again, but James is fearful of the man who has treated him so inconsistently in the past and rejects this idea. In the end, Graham and James commit themselves to living their lives as father and son thereafter, and they walk hand in hand through their town for the first time.

A third such movie is *Forrest Gump,* in which Robin Wright plays Jenny, Forrest's one true love throughout the decades. Jenny befriends Forrest as a child when none of the other children will, and their affection remains strong over the years, despite several long periods of separation. Although Jenny pursues romantic and sexual entanglements with several men over time, Forrest remains committed to her in his heart, and he passes up opportunities for sex with other women as a result. His greatest moments in life occur when he and Jenny are together "just like peas and carrots," and he longs for the day when Jenny will consent to being his wife. Ulti-mately she does, more than three years after she and Forrest share one night of sexual exploration and after she introduces him to their son. It is the early 1980s, and Jenny informs Forrest that she is sick with some kind of new and little understood virus that doctors presently cannot cure; the two wed shortly thereafter, with Forrest pledging always to take care of her and little Forrest. Jenny passes away quickly from AIDS, but Forrest's love for her remains strong ever after. He reminds her that he still loves her when visiting Jenny's grave, and that if she ever needs anything in the afterlife he will never be far away.

With regard to the representation of HIV/AIDS, the advantage that these three movies retain as compared to typical AIDS movies is that they "normalize" AIDS to a more significant degree, positioning the pandemic as a regular component of life in the modern age, while simultaneously reducing the otherness surrounding individuals confronting the disease. In an era in which the HIV/AIDS pandemic is directly affecting individuals of all kinds, the representation of AIDS characters in non-AIDS movies more effectively communicates the message that the AIDS threat surrounds all of us all of the time, and that social responses to AIDS require the involvement of myriad individuals, both personally infected and otherwise. In addition, unlike in so many AIDS movies, none of the AIDS characters in these three non-AIDS movies are explicitly represented to be gay men, serving to help break the persistent representational link between gay men and AIDS, thereby further reducing the otherness of AIDS and people with AIDS for the heterosexual majority of audience members.

The conclusion to Chapter 3 of this work emphasizes the need for the regular creation and dissemination of prosocial narratives about caring for others in their times of need—despite individual differences and despite the means by which they have contracted HIV/AIDS—and the non-AIDS movies discussed here all certainly achieve this goal. This alternative approach to representing AIDS may be especially beneficial to teenagers and young adults, who tend to reject the contents of movies that are overtly about AIDS because they are unable to personalize the risk that is being communicated in them, ultimately reinforcing their belief that AIDS is somebody else's problem (Kellar-Guenther, 1999, p. 218).

As AIDS researcher Yvonne Kellar-Guenther (1999, p. 218) has discovered, the message that HIV/AIDS is rampant in American society is not personalized by many young people today because it does not fit within their personal life experiences. Many young people do not yet personally know anybody living with HIV or anybody who has died from AIDS (Ibid.). If these young people choose not to expose themselves to typical AIDS movies because they cannot relate to the centrality of HIV/AIDS in them, it is presumed that they can still be reached with essential social information about the pandemic and their own risk of exposure through non-AIDS movies. Since these movies contain supporting characters with AIDS, they tend to soft-pedal their AIDS messages rather than beating viewers over the head with them.

Experts on AIDS education emphasize that because different audience members bring diverse personal histories and expectations to the viewing of any message about AIDS, offerings that contain multifaceted viewer appeals while simultaneously communicating information about HIV/AIDS hold the greatest potential to help change both the attitudes and the behaviors fostering the spread of HIV (Walters, Walters, and Priest, 1999, p. 304). In this regard, non-AIDS movies containing one or more AIDS characters may typically prove to be more effective than actual AIDS movies at retaining audience member interest among diverse audience members and subtly communicating much-needed social information about the current realities of the HIV/AIDS pandemic. Certainly, the inclusion of AIDS characters in non-AIDS movies such as the ones discussed here helps to counter the phenomenon of "invisible victims" (as discussed in Chapter 3), the many members of the general population who inaccurately believe that they are somehow shielded from infection with HIV/AIDS.

The enthusiasm generated in response to the inclusion of AIDS characters in the non-AIDS movies *Joey Breaker, Second Best,* and *Forrest Gump* is not meant to imply that the representations of AIDS characters in these offerings are not without their shortcomings, however. Although the character of Alfred is not explicitly encoded as a gay man in *Joey Breaker,* for example, his mannerisms and his former career as a librarian strongly suggest (stereotypically) that Alfred may indeed be gay. Similarly, although the character of John in *Second Best* never explicitly reveals how he contracted HIV/AIDS, the information that he has been in and out of prison repeatedly in recent years and the reality that he is never shown with nor discussing a woman strongly suggest (stereotypically) that he has become infected through man-to-man sexual activity in prison. As such, although these offerings do not explicitly link homosexuality and AIDS in their narratives, they nevertheless implicitly invoke this persistent representational link. Relatedly, although Forrest's undying devotion to Jenny in *Forrest Gump* is inspiring, and the movie's narrative never explicitly blames Jenny for her medical condition, all of the brief scenes featuring Jenny's "deviant ways" (her sexual promiscuity, her occasional drug use, her sexual involvement with an intravenous drug user in a hotel room, and the like) combine implicitly to blame her for contracting HIV/AIDS. In addition, none of these three representations of AIDS characters in non-AIDS movies does anything to alter the overreliance on featuring white characters, rather than characters from more diverse racial and ethnic backgrounds, as AIDS characters, despite the dramatic rates of HIV/AIDS transmission encountered in communities of color today. So although the representations of AIDS characters in these non-AIDS movies reflect differential degrees of progress in the representation of AIDS characters in movies, they nevertheless serve also as reminders of the amount of representational progress that has yet to be made.

Arguably, the most effective representation of an AIDS character in a non-AIDS movie, to date, occurs in the 1996 movie *Stealing Beauty,* a joint cinematic offering of Italy, France, and Great Britain, featuring American actress Liv Tyler, which received widespread theatrical distribution in the United States. In this movie, Jeremy Irons plays Alex Parrish, a successful playwright in the final stages of AIDS who lives out his remaining days among the company and support of artist friends at an Italian villa. When Lucy (played by Liv Tyler) arrives to spend the summer searching for her biological father, she befriends Alex, and they spend many hours together talking about their lives, smoking pot, taking long walks, and gossiping about the others. Although Lucy is consumed with her search and with her desire to lose her virginity, she nevertheless becomes protective of Alex, checking in on him regularly and watching over him at night as he sleeps. In turn, Alex tends to an injury Lucy obtains while bicycling and helps her to discover her dreams and desires. Near the end of the movie, when Alex's health has declined further and he must be taken to a hospital to ease his pain during the final days of his life, Lucy sends him off with a good-bye kiss on the lips, an extended hug, and a marijuana cigarette for him to share with the nurses. Fulfilling the quests she began under Alex's guidance, Lucy succeeds in locating her biological father, finding the true love of her life, and losing her virginity by firelight in a romantic setting.

What is most impressive about the representation of Alex as an AIDS character in the non-AIDS movie *Stealing Beauty* is that (1) he is encoded to be a heterosexual male, (2) the mode by which he contracted HIV/AIDS is never made explicit in the narrative, (3) nobody either explicitly or implicitly blames Alex for his infection with HIV/AIDS, and (4) everybody treats Alex the same way they treat everybody else in their social world, showing compassion for his emotional and physical needs, while treating his AIDS status as simply another part of his personal history. Such a representation goes a long way toward eradicating the culturally shared distancing formula that produces the perception that AIDS happens to somebody else—presumably gay men and intravenous drug users—a perception that inaccurately prevents many individuals from considering themselves to be at risk of contracting HIV/AIDS. It serves as an alternate, more unique way of "humanizing" the AIDS pandemic that more accurately reflects the cumulative impact of HIV/AIDS on individuals throughout the world.

AIDS METAPHOR MOVIES

A variation on including AIDS characters in non-AIDS movies involves featuring characters with symptoms similar to those of HIV/AIDS in non-AIDS movies that are encoded intentionally to serve as metaphors for AIDS movies. In other words, the narratives of AIDS metaphor movies do not explicitly incorporate characters living with and/or dying from HIV/AIDS specifically; rather, they incorporate characters living with and/or dying from medical conditions that are metaphorically analogous to HIV/AIDS.

The most straightforward example of this process occurs in the 1993 movie *Daybreak*, which features Cuba Gooding Jr. as Torch, the African-American leader of a group of resistance fighters who seek to free disease-infected individuals from ultimate quarantine in isolation camps. The narrative unfolds in New York City during the early decades of the new millennium, at a time when a nameless, sexually transmitted epidemic is spreading across America. The government requires quarterly testing of all Americans, who are classified as "negatives" and "positives." While negatives are allowed to go about their daily lives freely, positives are tattooed with a P on their chests, which enables them to be tracked constantly by radar. Positives are also quarantined in dismal locations, to safeguard the health and security of the majority of negatives. After Torch is apprehended by government officials and determined to be a positive, his girlfriend, Blue (played by Moira Kelly), a negative, sneaks into the location where he is being confined and attempts to engage in unprotected sex with him so that she can become a positive and the two can live out their final days together. Torch, however, refuses to be responsible for her death over time and sends her off to lead the resistance in his absence.

Clearly, from start to finish, the narrative of *Daybreak* is intentionally constructed to serve as a metaphor for the AIDS pandemic. By focusing explicitly on a nameless disease rather than HIV/AIDS specifically, it enables (and encourages) viewers to contemplate complex issues surrounding the social construction of, and social reactions to, infectious diseases such as AIDS in American society, including the most desirable level of interaction between infected individuals and the general population as well as the related alternatives of quarantine and physical identification of the unhealthy. All of these issues surfaced during the early years of the AIDS pandemic, and their introduction into AIDS metaphor movies more fully enables viewers to assess the validity of various alternatives more objectively, without the associated context of fear and discrimination that pervaded American society in the years following the discovery of HIV/AIDS.

Another positive aspect of the metaphoric representation of AIDS in *Daybreak* is the movie's regular portrayal of women and people of color—rather than gay men or drug injectors—as being at risk for this sexually transmitted disease. As such, this representation effectively evokes the anxieties generated by the AIDS pandemic, without subjecting its viewers to more stereotypical portrayals of infected homosexuals and drug addicts (Goldstein, 1991, p. 22). This potentially increases the homophily (defined as degree of similarity) between the movie's characters and its viewers, thereby expanding the social construction of AIDS as a disease that regularly affects all kinds of Americans—at least among those viewers who recognize that this movie is designed to serve as a metaphor for AIDS.

Similar metaphoric representations of AIDS occur in the movies *Safe* (1995) and *Prelude to a Kiss* (1992). Although not as readily identifiable as an AIDS metaphor movie as is *Daybreak, Safe* features actress Julianne Moore as Carol, a Southern California housewife whose health becomes compromised by unseen harmful invaders that doctors cannot seem to identify. With each passing day, Carol becomes increasingly allergic to her surrounding world. Her body's immune system is no longer able to fend off the "harmless" effects of pesticides, exhaust fumes, and various chemicals (such as those found in hair-care products) encountered in everyday life at the end of the twentieth century. Although she suffers from fatigue, nosebleeds, vomiting spells, and seizures, Carol's doctor insists that he cannot find anything wrong with her and assures her that she is "perfectly healthy." She then leaves her husband and stepson behind and seeks relief at a New Age holistic health center in the desert, where a self-appointed "expert" on sufferers of "environmental illness" persuades clients that they can heal themselves simply by learning to love themselves. Although she still becomes physically ill when exposed to fumes of various kinds, Carol convinces herself that she did indeed become ill because she hated herself, before she retreated to the desert, and that the cure for her condition lies in learning to love herself again. The movie thus ends with images of Carol speaking the words "I love you" to her reflection in a mirror.

Safe suggests early on that Carol's compromised health condition may somehow be the result of unprotected sexual intercourse with her husband, with whom she is shown having sex during the first few minutes of the movie. This is the first hint to the viewer that this movie is being constructed as a metaphor for AIDS. Less than five minutes later, Carol learns that a friend's brother has died suddenly, and that because the man was unmarried, everyone jumps to the same conclusion about his cause of death. This discussion also brings the topic of AIDS to the mind of the viewer, even though it is never explicitly mentioned.

Viewers who fail to pick up on these initial references to AIDS, however, may still catch on to the metaphoric status of this narrative if they have a solid understanding of the social history of HIV/ AIDS in American society, such as the reality that, during the pandemic's early years, various social actors blamed the compromised health conditions of people with AIDS on the self-loathing of those infected. Those viewers who ultimately recognize *Safe* to be an intentional metaphor for HIV/AIDS infection are able to explore more fully the fears and frustrations associated with having an unknown, emerging medical condition, as well as the absurdity of blaming victims of infectious diseases for their unfortunate health outcomes, in a way that is somewhat detached from the social and historical realities of HIV/AIDS and, therefore, potentially more objective. Unfortunately, such a desirable end result is lost on viewers who fail to recognize the metaphoric status of a movie such as *Safe,* which represents a potentially significant overall shortcoming of AIDS metaphor movies.

To an even greater extent than with *Safe,* many viewers of *Prelude to a Kiss* likely never even recognize that it is intentionally encoded to serve as an AIDS metaphor movie, unless they were informed of this fact through widespread reports in the gay press at the time the movie premiered in theaters nationwide. In this movie, Alec Baldwin and Meg Ryan star as Peter and Rita, a young couple who fall in love and decide to marry. On the day of their wedding, Rita is kissed by an unknown old man; in the process, the souls of Rita and the old man become transposed, and Rita gradually transforms from a healthy, energetic bride into a sickly, dying one. When it is revealed that Rita has less than one year left to live, Peter launches a successful plan to reunite Rita and the old man and, through another kiss and a mutual desire by the two to switch souls once again, restore his bride to her original healthy, youthful self. The moral of the story, as explained by Peter at movie's end, is that the miracle of another living human being must never be squandered.

Similar to *Daybreak* and *Safe, Prelude to a Kiss* contains its share of clues to the viewer that it is intended to serve as an AIDS metaphor movie. Early conversations between Peter and Rita focus on her clean bill of health when they first meet (despite her insomnia) and the use of protection during sex. The kiss between Rita and the old man is intended to signify an act of unprotected, casual sex. A strange conversation between Peter and his best friend involves

Peter talking about strangers "going inside" one another (presumably to switch souls) and is concluded by his friend inquiring as to why somebody would want to go inside the body of another person whom he or she does not really know. Finally, the entire plot of someone's health status changing dramatically right before the eyes of another further suggests the metaphoric quality of this work. The only problem is that many viewers will fail to fully comprehend the significance of these clues, which suggests that they will also miss out on the metaphoric significance of the entire work and its corresponding intended message.

When AIDS metaphor movies (such as *Daybreak*) can readily be identified as such by their viewers and are reflected upon accordingly, they hold tremendous potential to further "normalize" AIDS as a disease that affects all kinds of Americans and to eradicate the widely shared misperception that HIV/AIDS is a concern of "the other" rather than of the self. At the same time, they regularly challenge the social construction of AIDS as a "gay disease" and enable many Americans to contemplate more fully the impact of HIV/AIDS on all of American society and on individuals throughout the world. The only problem with some AIDS metaphor movies is that, in their attempts to be intellectually stimulating and a bit more narratively complex than more straightforward narratives, their desired effects on viewers may never be achieved; many viewers may fail to identify the metaphoric link between the movies' explicit contents and their intended implicit associations and, therefore, will fail to question their existing, socially shared construction of the AIDS pandemic. Such offerings must therefore be considered to be potentially powerful representational assets in the quest to alter and expand the social construction of HIV/AIDS in American society, ones capable of significant ends in the skilled hands of individuals who fully understand how most effectively to utilize the representational means at their disposal.

SELF-REPRESENTATION IN AIDS DOCUMENTARIES

Yet another way of representing AIDS in movies involves the featuring of actual people with AIDS in AIDS documentaries that are created through their direct participation. From time to time, individuals living with and/or dying from AIDS choose to make documentaries about their experiences with assistance from their lovers, friends, and trusted associates, for ultimate presentation to viewers nationwide. These films are made in an attempt to more realistically depict conditions encountered by people in the final stages of AIDS and to reinforce the importance of all individuals protecting themselves consistently from the risks of the pandemic as they go about their daily lives. In contrast to the numerous documentaries about AIDS that have been made over the past two decades by cultural "outsiders" depicting people other than themselves or communities other than their own, this distinctive subset of AIDS documentaries offers a form of alternative representational production, involving the creation of images from within the community of individuals who are living with and/or dying from AIDS (Juhasz, 1998, pp. 206-207). The resulting creations tend to have far lower production values than the other kinds of movies about AIDS discussed in this project, which contributes significantly to perceptions of their greater "authenticity" with regard to the realistic representation of HIV/AIDS in American society. Three of the most widely available documentaries of this kind are *Silverlake Life: The View from Here* (1993); *Fast Trip, Long Drop* (1994); and *Life and Death on the A-List* (1996).

By far, the best-known example of self-representation in an AIDS documentary occurs in *Silverlake Life: The View from Here,* a video diary begun by Los Angeles filmmaker Tom Joslin after his gay lover of more than two decades, Mark Massi, was diagnosed with AIDS in 1989. Soon after, when Joslin's own battle with AIDS accelerated more quickly than Massi's, the focus of the project shifted painfully to recording the health decline and death of Joslin himself, with Massi assuming more of the shooting responsibilities over time (Seckinger and Jakobsen, 1997, p. 145). The efforts of Joslin and Massi were supplemented by the camera work of several of their friends, as well as by the editing of Peter Friedman, one of Joslin's former film students, who spent fifteen months completing the project and transferring it to 16 millimeter (mm) film for national distribution after Massi's death in 1991 (Ibid.).

The "authentic" aura of this documentary is established immediately from its opening shots of Joslin and Massi in their Silverlake home, which are shaky and not properly white-balanced,* and therefore readily interpreted as being the work of "ordinary people" rather than "professionals." Within minutes, the viewer is confronted with visuals and dialogue pertaining to unpleasant medical procedures, unique forms of therapy, and graphic glimpses into what it is really like to be living with AIDS. During one such graphic glimpse, Joslin (speaking directly to the camera) explains how even the simplest five-minute task out in public sends him back to his vehicle to lie down; in another, he explains how his doctor described the form of AIDS-related brain disease that he suffers from as being similar to bats hanging upside down from the back of a person's brain stem and gradually eating their way to the top. Just ten minutes into *Silverlake Life*, the degree to which this representation of HIV/AIDS differs from the more sanitized fictional versions becomes remarkably clear to the viewer. As the work continues, the viewer is offered realistic glimpses of the deep love and caring that is evident between these two gay men, in the form of loving glances, good-night kisses, and discussions of how one cannot imagine having to live without the other. The viewer is also confronted with continuous glimpses into the fear, fatigue, frustration, and sense of isolation that typically accompany living with AIDS, such as during a sequence in which Joslin awakens in the middle of the night in pain and turns on a flashlight and the video camera to record the depths of his discomfort, or when he begins speaking of events that have never occurred, as his condition worsens.

The most memorable, moving, and simultaneously disconcerting sequence in *Silverlake Life* occurs more than an hour into the documentary, just minutes after Joslin has died of AIDS. Massi focuses the camera on Joslin's lifeless face and, while attempting to fight back his own tears, sings "You Are My Sunshine" to his dead lover, the way he did just minutes before at the moment of Joslin's passing. Commenting on Joslin's beauty even in death, Massi promises to

---

*"White-balancing" is the procedure followed by videographers to properly adjust their video cameras to various lighting conditions, to ensure that objects that are white in reality also appear that way on video (rather than yellowish, greenish, etc.). Videographers must white-balance their cameras any time lighting conditions change, such as when moving from indoors to outdoors.

Joslin that all of his friends will finish the documentary for him. Seconds later, after Massi has bid farewell to Joslin, he pulls back the sheet covering Joslin's emaciated body, vividly revealing the devastating physical consequences experienced by individuals living with and dying from AIDS. The remainder of the documentary focuses on Massi's attempts to manage the complex emotions he encounters following the death of the man he loved so greatly. At the time of its release, *Silverlake Life* was widely considered to be one of the most in-depth portraits of living with and dying from AIDS ever to be seen by a large, typically underinformed audience (Seckinger and Jakobsen, 1997, p. 146). Today, the representation of HIV/AIDS in this work still serves as a dramatic reminder of how rarely the American public is exposed to the realistic articulation of such perseverance and pain in other kinds of media representations of AIDS (Ibid., p. 144).

In much the same way as *Silverlake Life, Life and Death on the A-List* painfully and realistically portrays the complications of living with AIDS in American society. What distinguishes this work most greatly from *Silverlake Life,* however, is that its subject is a somewhat better-known American "celebrity": the ruggedly handsome, gay actor and model Tom McBride, who is perhaps best remembered for his appearances in Winston cigarette ads and as the dancing Dr. Pepper man. As he became increasingly sick and debilitated from AIDS, McBride asked his friend and fellow actor Jay Corcoran to videotape the final months of his life. The resulting documentary captures the pain experienced by a member of the New York City "A-list crowd" who falls from grace in the eyes of others in that social circle as a result of losing his looks and his hard body due to his declining health. At the same time, it offers glimpses into the lifestyle, past and present, of an attractive gay man who remains unapologetic about the pleasures he derived from sex with numerous attractive men. The viewer is presented with candid insights into the dynamics of "fucking" and "being fucked" as a member of the gay community, as well as the potential negative ramifications of such unprotected practices, vividly reinforced with disturbing visual images of McBride becoming progressively disabled by AIDS and wasting away in his (death)bed, no longer able to speak.

As in *Silverlake Life* and *Life and Death on the A-List,* the documentary *Fast Trip, Long Drop* features images and dialogue of an individual confronting the complexities associated with living with HIV/AIDS in the United States. In this instance, that individual is videographer and AIDS activist Gregg Bordowitz, who considers himself to have a gay identity (rather than a bisexual one), even though he has engaged in sexual relations with both men and women over time. This documentary contains similarly powerful images of the fears and frustrations that typically accompany everyday life with AIDS, taking the viewer to an AIDS support group meeting, at which participants contemplate ways to remain hopeful in the face of increasing loss; to gatherings for AIDS activism, with their increasing air of disillusion as the pandemic continues; and into the homes of family members who fear losing loved ones far too soon. What most significantly distinguishes this documentary from the previous two, however, is that it intersperses brief scripted, performed critiques of typical representations of HIV/AIDS in American society throughout the documentary footage, to produce a more richly layered, multivalent perspective on living with and dying from AIDS (Seckinger and Jakobsen, 1997, p. 154). During such critiques, Bordowitz and a few of his associates assume the roles of a homophobic news anchor, an uncaring counselor, a heterosexual "innocent victim," and related (stereotypic) others to explore more fully the ways in which people with AIDS—and gay men especially—are regularly treated negatively in American society. Although this documentary could proceed effectively without them, such critiques serve primarily to strengthen the impact of the contents of their surrounding documentary images by more blatantly calling into question the typical functioning of media professionals, health care professionals, government officials, and other influential social actors in response to the AIDS pandemic.

Certainly, one great strength of self-representation of people with AIDS in documentaries such as these is that the resulting creations avoid the historical approach common to most documentaries, which tend to focus on "society's victims" and turn their subjects into "media victims" as well, by exploiting "deviance" to titillate viewers (Seckinger and Jakobsen, 1997, p. 150). Such a process frequently occurs whenever the documentary subject is cast as "the other," someone considered to be socially separate from the documentary makers, who retain control over the ultimate representation of that subject (Ibid.). Self-representation in the documentaries discussed here serves to collapse the roles of documentary maker and subject, helping to ensure that the resulting representation of HIV/AIDS is a more informed and better balanced one. Media studies scholar Alexandra Juhasz quite eloquently summarizes this state of affairs when she explains, "A most significant way in which alternative videomaking—usually work produced for little expense and with little formal training using camcorders and other inexpensive or low-end video technologies—counters and alters mainstream media is that it localizes the production and reception of this usually universalizing mode of discourse" (1998, p. 206). Accordingly, self-representation in AIDS documentaries provides increased opportunities for expanding the social construction of what various kinds of people with AIDS are actually like.

Another significant strength of self-representation in AIDS documentaries is that the resulting creations feature real people experiencing real situations (rather than fictional characters encountering fictional situations), thereby heightening their overall emotional and social impact on many viewers. Although each of the AIDS documentaries discussed here is necessarily a form of subjective interpretation rather than "objective reality," all of them derive their claim of being "truthful" precisely as a result of their being fundamentally interpretive (Hamilton, 1997, p. 146). In other words, it is precisely because the images depicted in these documentaries are so intimately tied to the personal experiences and interpretations of the individuals choosing to capture them that they appear to lay claim to a wider truth about HIV/AIDS and achieve a more solid sense of representational legitimacy than fictional representations allow (Ibid., pp. 146-147). The association of the videographer's intimate interpretive grasp of his or her subject matter combined with the seemingly objective video image secures a privileged status for these documentaries that exceeds the status afforded by viewers to fictional representations of AIDS in movies (Ibid, p. 147).

Despite their representational advantages, however, the major potential shortcoming of these documentaries lies in the fact that they are, indeed, documentaries, a type of media offering that is disfavored by many viewers in the modern age. Although American viewers in recent years have demonstrated a desire for documentary images of real-life situations with regard to sensationalistic "news" programs and real-life action programs such as *Cops,* this enthusiasm does not always translate into a corresponding desire for more traditional, full-length documentaries such as the ones discussed here, especially when they focus on disconcerting topics such as AIDS (Seckinger and Jakobsen, 1997, p. 154).

THE (NEAR) FUTURE OF REPRESENTING AIDS

An article about the present state of HIV/AIDS in the March 1999 issue of *Esquire* magazine begins, "We thought the worst epidemic in history had been subdued. But this is not the same AIDS. This is a monster that is mutating faster than we can keep up. It's alive. It's healthy. And the worst is yet to come" (Garrett, 1999, p. 103).

Unfortunately, as those words suggest, claims that a cure for AIDS had been found in the form of drug combination "cocktails" and that the eradication of HIV/AIDS was at hand—which reached the height of their fervor in the United States during the period between summer 1996 and spring 1998—have proven to be quite premature, as failures of such therapies have since been occurring regularly in individuals infected with HIV/AIDS (Greene and Cassidy, 1999, p. 369; Garrett, 1999, p. 104). Although the AIDS death rate in the United States decreased by 47 percent between 1996 and 1997, it has since begun to rise again, and the rate of new infection has not decreased (Ibid., p. 105; Wheeler, 1999, p. A21). Rather than being eradicated, HIV hid for awhile, mutated, and rebounded with a renewed vengeance. As the seventeen-year-old pandemic continues to infect 16,000 new individuals around the world daily, neither a cure nor a vaccine is in sight (Garrett, 1999, p. 106; Wheeler, 1999, p. A21).

Dr. Mathilde Krim, cofounder and chairperson of the American Foundation for AIDS Research, explains that the American public has vastly overinterpreted the positive strides made in the fight against AIDS over the past two decades, to the point that Americans feel that HIV/AIDS is no longer much of a concern (*Esquire*, 1999,

p. 109). She cautions that if Americans do not continue to respond in responsible ways to the threat of contracting HIV/AIDS over the next ten years, the United States may find itself, a decade from now, facing the same grave situation from AIDS that the continent of Africa is facing today (Ibid.).

Today, at the start of the third decade of HIV/AIDS, the need for diverse and more accurate representations of AIDS in movies and other media offerings has never been greater. Today, when new infection rates among gay white men in American society (and throughout North America) continue to decline while infection rates among members of other social groups—especially women, minorities, and adolescents—continue to rise, these representations must reach the estimated one-third of all Americans who are HIV positive yet do not know it (Garrett, 1999, p. 172).They also must reach the millions of Americans who are still HIV negative and wish to remain that way. The need for unique ways to represent AIDS that will reach these groups has never been more severe.

As communication scholars Nancy Roth and Linda Fuller have emphasized:

> In the absence of a cure or vaccine, communication is central to efforts to stem the spread of the HIV virus and to care for those who are already infected. The ways that HIV and those infected and affected by the virus are constructed, communicatively, affects transmission/prevention, caregiver-patient relationships, and media outcomes. Media representations play a large role in popular perceptions of the disease and those infected and affected by it. (1998, p. 2)

Well into the next decade of the AIDS pandemic and (likely) beyond, AIDS movies, AIDS metaphor movies, AIDS documentaries, and related ways of representing AIDS can serve as powerful forces in influencing the ongoing social construction and reconstruction of the pandemic and the individuals who perceive themselves to be at risk for infection or transmission. The secret to success lies in identifying and learning from the shortcomings common to representations of AIDS and people with AIDS in media offerings, past and present, to provide even more effective representations that can help stem the tide of the pandemic in the coming years.

Appendix A

Complete List of AIDS Movies Compiled

And the Band Played On (1993, Roger Spottiswoode)
Andre's Mother (1990, Deborah Reinisch)
As Is (1986, Michael Lindsay-Hogg)
Boys on the Side (1994, Herbert Ross)
Breaking the Surface: The Greg Louganis Story (1996, Steven Hilliard Stern)
Buddies (1985, Arthur J. Bressan Jr.)
Chain of Desire (1992, Temistocles Lopez)
Chocolate Babies (1996, Stephen Winter)
Citizen Cohn (1992, Frank Pierson)
The Cure (1995, Peter Horton)
An Early Frost (1985, John Erman)
Gia (1998, Michael Cristofer)
Go Toward the Light (1988, Mike Robe)
Grief (1993, Richard Glatzer)
The Immortals (1995, Brian Grant)
In the Gloaming (1997, Christopher Reeve)
It's My Party (1996, Randal Kleiser)
Jeffrey (1995, Christopher Ashley)
Jerker (1991, Hugh Harrison)
Kids (1995, Larry Clark)
The Littlest Victims (1989, Peter Levin)
The Living End (1992, Gregg Araki)
Longtime Companion (1990, Norman Rene)
Love! Valour! Compassion! (1997, Joe Mantello)
Men in Love (1989, Marc Huestis)
A Mother's Prayer (1995, Larry Elikann)
My Brother's Keeper (1995, Glenn Jordan)
On Common Ground (1992, Hugh Harrison)
One Night Stand (1997, Mike Figgis)
Our Sons (1991, John Erman)

Parting Glances (1986, Bill Sherwood)
Philadelphia (1993, Jonathan Demme)
A Place for Annie (1994, John Gray)
Red Ribbon Blues (1995, Charles Winkler)
Roommates (1994, Alan Metzger)
The Ryan White Story (1989, John Herzfeld)
Something to Live For: The Alison Gertz Story (1992, Tim
    McLoughlin)
Tidy Endings (1988, Gavin Millar)
Under Heat (1994, Peter Reed)
World and Time Enough (1995, Eric Mueller)

Appendix B

List of AIDS Movies
Analyzed in This Study

And the Band Played On (1993, Roger Spottiswoode)
As Is (1986, Michael Lindsay-Hogg)
Boys on the Side (1994, Herbert Ross)
Breaking the Surface: The Greg Louganis Story (1996, Steven Hilliard Stern)
Chain of Desire (1992, Temistocles Lopez)
Chocolate Babies (1996, Stephen Winter)
Citizen Cohn (1992, Frank Pierson)
The Cure (1995, Peter Horton)
An Early Frost (1985, John Erman)
Gia (1998, Michael Cristofer)
Grief (1993, Richard Glatzer)
The Immortals (1995, Brian Grant)
In the Gloaming (1997, Christopher Reeve)
It's My Party (1996, Randal Kleiser)
Jeffrey (1995, Christopher Ashley)
Jerker (1991, Hugh Harrison)
Kids (1995, Larry Clark)
The Living End (1992, Gregg Araki)
Longtime Companion (1990, Norman Rene)
Love! Valour! Compassion! (1997, Joe Mantello)
Men in Love (1989, Marc Huestis)
A Mother's Prayer (1995, Larry Elikann)
On Common Ground (1992, Hugh Harrison)
One Night Stand (1997, Mike Figgis)
Our Sons (1991, John Erman)
Parting Glances (1986, Bill Sherwood)
Philadelphia (1993, Jonathan Demme)
A Place for Annie (1994, John Gray)

The Ryan White Story (1989, John Herzfeld)
Something to Live For: The Alison Gertz Story (1992, Tim
   McLoughlin)
Under Heat (1994, Peter Reed)
World and Time Enough (1995, Eric Mueller)

References

Altman, Dennis. *The Homosexualization of America.* New York: St. Martin's Press, 1982.

Beaver, Frank. *Dictionary of Film Terms: The Aesthetic Companion to Film Analysis.* New York: Twayne Publishers, 1994.

Belton, John. *American Cinema/American Culture.* New York: McGraw-Hill, 1994.

Between the Lines. "Health News: AIDS on Rise in Young Gay Men." *Between the Lines,* February 3 (1999): 18.

Between the Lines. "Young People Underestimate AIDS." *Between the Lines,* January 7 (1999): 17.

Britton, Andrew. "Blissing Out: The Politics of Reaganite Entertainment." *Movie* 31/32 (Winter, 1986): 1-42.

Byars, Jackie. *All That Hollywood Allows: Re-Reading Gender in 1950s Melodrama.* Chapel Hill, NC: University of North Carolina Press, 1991.

Cadwell, Steve. "Twice Removed: The Stigma Suffered by Gay Men with AIDS." *Smith College Studies in Social Work* 61(3) (1991): 236-246.

Cathcart, Robert. "The *Guiding Light:* Soap Opera As Economic Product and Cultural Document." In *Intermedia: Interpersonal Communication in a Media World,* Eds. Gary Gumpert and Robert Cathcart. New York: Oxford University Press, 1986, pp. 207-218.

Clark, Kevin A. "Pink Water: The Archetype of Blood and the Pool of Infinite Contagion." In *Power in the Blood: A Handbook on AIDS, Politics, and Communication,* Ed. William N. Elwood. Mahwah, NJ: Lawrence Erlbaum Associates, 1999, pp. 9-24.

Clarke, David B., Ed. *The Cinematic City.* New York: Routledge, 1997.

Collins, Jim. "Genericity in the Nineties: Eclectic Irony and the New Sincerity." In *Film Theory Goes to the Movies,* Eds. Jim Collins, Hilary Radner, and Ava Preacher Collins. New York: Routledge, 1993, pp. 242-263.

Cook, Timothy E. and David C. Colby. "The Mass-Mediated Epidemic: The Politics of AIDS on the Nightly Network News." In *AIDS: The Making of a Chronic Disease,* Eds. Elizabeth Fee and Daniel M. Fox. Berkeley, CA: University of California Press, 1992, pp. 84-122.

Crimp, Douglas. "AIDS: Cultural Analysis/Cultural Activism." *October* (43) (1987): 3-16.

Croteau, James M. and Susanne Morgan. "Combating Homophobia in AIDS Education." *Journal of Counseling and Development* 68(1) (1989): 86-91.

Dyer, Richard, Ed. *The Matter of Images: Essays on Representation.* New York: Routledge, 1993.

Easthope, Antony. "Cinecities in the Sixties." In *The Cinematic City,* Ed. David B. Clarke. New York: Routledge, 1997, pp. 129-139.

Elwood, William N., Ed. *Power in the Blood: A Handbook on AIDS, Politics, and Communication.* Mahwah, NJ: Lawrence Erlbaum Associates, 1999.

Erni, John Nguyet. *Unstable Frontiers: Technomedicine and the Cultural Politics of "Curing" AIDS.* Minneapolis, MN: Minnesota University Press, 1994.

Esquire. "Why We're Here," *Esquire* 131(3) (March 1999): 108-109.

Estrada, Antonio and Gilbert A. Quintero. "Redefining Categories of Risk and Identity: The Appropriation of AIDS Prevention Information and Constructions of Risk." In *Power in the Blood: A Handbook on AIDS, Politics, and Communication,* Ed. William N. Elwood. Mahwah, NJ: Lawrence Erlbaum Associates, 1999, pp. 133-147.

Farber, Stephen. "A Drama of Family Loyalty, Acceptance—and AIDS." *The New York Times,* August 18 (1985): 23+.

Fee, Elizabeth and Daniel M. Fox, Eds. *AIDS: The Making of a Chronic Disease.* Berkeley, CA: University of California Press, 1992.

Gamson, Joshua. "Silence, Death, and the Invisible Enemy: AIDS Activism and Social Movement 'Newness.' " *Social Problems* 36(4) (1989): 351-367.

Garrett, Laurie. "The Virus at the End of the World." *Esquire* 131(3) (March 1999): 102-107+.

GLAAD Images. "GLAAD Dives into USA Network with *Breaking the Surface.*" *GLAAD Images* (Spring 1997): 4.

Goldstein, Richard. "The Implicated and the Immune: Responses to AIDS in the Arts and Popular Culture." In *A Disease of Society: Cultural and Institutional Responses to AIDS,* Eds. Dorothy Nelkin, David P. Willis, and Scott V. Parris. Cambridge: Cambridge University Press, 1991, pp. 17-42.

Gollin, Richard M. *A Viewer's Guide to Film.* New York: McGraw-Hill, 1992.

Green/Epstein Productions. "The Making of *Breaking the Surface: The Greg Louganis Story.*" Online (1997). Available <http://www.breaksurf.com/making.htm>.

Greene, Kathryn and Barbara Cassidy. "Ethical Choices Regarding Noncompliance: Prescribing Protease Inhibitors for HIV-Infected Female Adolescents." In *Power in the Blood: A Handbook on AIDS, Politics, and Communication,* Ed. William N. Elwood. Mahwah, NJ: Lawrence Erlbaum Associates, 1999, pp. 369-384.

Gross, Larry. "What Is Wrong with This Picture? Lesbian Women and Gay Men on Television." In *Queer Words, Queer Images: Communication and the Construction of Homosexuality,* Ed. R. Jeffrey Ringer. New York: New York University Press, 1994, pp. 143-156.

Grover, Jan Zita. "AIDS: Keywords." In *AIDS: Cultural Analysis, Cultural Activism,* Ed. Douglas Crimp. Cambridge, MA: MIT Press, 1987, pp. 17-31.

Hall, Stuart. "The Rediscovery of 'Ideology': Return of the Repressed in Media Studies." In *Culture, Society, and the Media,* Ed. Michael Gurevitch. London: Methuen, 1982, pp. 56-90.

Hall, Stuart. "The Spectacle of the 'Other.' " *Representation: Cultural Representations and Signifying Practices,* Ed. Stuart Hall. Thousand Oaks, CA: Sage, 1997, pp. 223-279.

Hamilton, Peter. "Representing the Social: France and Frenchness in Post-War Humanist Photography." In *Representation: Cultural Representations and Signifying Practices*, Ed. Stuart Hall. Thousand Oaks, CA: Sage, 1997, pp. 75-150.

Hart, Kylo-Patrick R. "Representation of AIDS on *Beverly Hills 90210:* Theoretical Concerns and Focus Group Findings." Ninth Annual Meeting of the Far West Popular Culture and Far West American Culture Associations. Imperial Palace Hotel, Las Vegas, February 1, 1997.

Hart, Kylo-Patrick R. "Retrograde Representation: The Lone Gay White Male Dying of AIDS on *Beverly Hills, 90210.*" *The Journal of Men's Studies* 7(2) (1999): 201-213.

Hayward, Susan. *Key Concepts in Cinema Studies*. New York: Routledge, 1996.

Herek, Gregory M. "The Social Context of Hate Crimes: Notes on Cultural Heterosexism." In *Hate Crimes: Confronting Violence Against Lesbians and Gay Men*, Eds. Gregory M. Herek and K. Berril. Newbury Park, CA: Sage Publications, 1992, pp. 89-104.

Herek, Gregory M. and Eric K. Glunt. "An Epidemic of Stigma: Public Reactions to AIDS." *American Psychologist* 43(11) (1988): 886-891.

Hogan, Katie. "Gendered Visibilities in Black Women's AIDS Narratives." In *Gendered Epidemic: Representations of Women in the Age of AIDS*, Eds. Nancy L. Roth and Katie Hogan. New York: Routledge, 1998, pp. 165-190.

Juhasz, Alexandra. "Make a Video for Me." In *Gendered Epidemic: Representations of Women in the Age of AIDS*, Eds. Nancy L. Roth and Katie Hogan. New York: Routledge, 1998, pp. 205-220.

Kellar-Guenther, Yvonne. "The Power of Romance: Changing the Focus of AIDS Education Messages." In *Power in the Blood: A Handbook on AIDS, Politics, and Communication*, Ed. William N. Elwood. Mahwah, NJ: Lawrence Erlbaum Associates, 1999, pp. 215-229.

Klaprat, Cathy. "The Star As Market Strategy: Bette Davis in Another Light." In *The American Film Industry*, Ed. Tino Balio. Madison, WI: University of Wisconsin Press, 1985, pp. 351-376.

Landy, Marcia, Ed. *Imitations of Life: A Reader on Film and Television Melodrama*. Detroit, MI: Wayne State University Press, 1991.

Lang, Robert. *American Film Melodrama*. Princeton: Princeton University Press, 1989.

Lopez, Daniel. *Films by Genre*. London: McFarland and Company, 1993.

Mahoney, Elisabeth. " 'The People in Parentheses': Space Under Pressure in the Postmodern City." In *The Cinematic City*, Ed. David B. Clarke. New York: Routledge, 1997, pp. 168-185.

Maltby, Richard. *Hollywood Cinema*. Cambridge, MA: Blackwell Publishers, 1995.

McArthur, Colin. "Chinese Boxes and Russian Dolls: Tracking the Elusive Cinematic City." In *The Cinematic City*, Ed. David B. Clarke. New York: Routledge, 1997, pp. 19-45.

McCoy, Clyde B., Christine Miles, and Lisa R. Metsch. "The Medicalization of Discourse Within an AIDS Research Setting." In *Power in the Blood: A Hand-*

book on AIDS, Politics, and Communication, Ed. William N. Elwood. Mahwah, NJ: Lawrence Erlbaum Associates, 1999, pp. 39-50.

McKinney, Mitchell S. and Bryan G. Pepper. "From Hope to Heartbreak: Bill
Clinton and the Rhetoric of AIDS." In *Power in the Blood: A Handbook on
AIDS, Politics, and Communication*, Ed. William N. Elwood. Mahwah, NJ:
Lawrence Erlbaum Associates, 1999, pp. 77-92.

Millman, Doreen. "Remarks from the Opening Ceremony of the XI International
Conference on AIDS." *The Daily Progress,* July 8 (1996): 1, 3.

Morse, Stephen S. "AIDS and Beyond: Defining the Rules for Viral Traffic." In
AIDS: The Making of a Chronic Disease, Eds. Elizabeth Fee and Daniel M.
Fox. Berkeley, CA: University of California Press, 1992, pp. 23-48.

Nelson, Victoria S. "The Reagan Administration's Response to AIDS: Conservative Argument and Conflict." In *Power in the Blood: A Handbook on AIDS,
Politics, and Communication*, Ed. William N. Elwood. Mahwah, NJ: Lawrence Erlbaum Associates, 1999, pp. 53-66.

Netzhammer, Emile C. and Scott A. Shamp. "Guilt by Association: Homosexual-
ity and AIDS on Prime-Time Television." In *Queer Words, Queer Images:
Communication and the Construction of Homosexuality*, Ed. R. Jeffrey Ringer.
New York: New York University Press, 1994.

Out Post. "AIDS Advisory Chair: Don't Be Fooled by Death Decline." *Out Post,*
May 27 (1998): 11.

Padgug, Robert A. and Gerald M. Oppenheimer. "Riding the Tiger: AIDS and the
Gay Community." In *AIDS: The Making of a Chronic Disease*, Eds. Elizabeth
Fee and Daniel M. Fox. Berkeley, CA: University of California Press, 1992,
pp. 245-278.

Parish, James R. and Michael R. Pitts. *The Great Science Fiction Pictures.* Metu-
chen, NJ: The Scarecrow Press, Inc., 1977.

Patton, Cindy. *Inventing AIDS*. New York: Routledge, 1990.

Perrow, Charles and Mauro F. Guillen. *The AIDS Disaster: The Failure of Organizations in New York and the Nation*. New Haven, CT: Yale University Press,
1990.

Pilipp, Frank and Charles Shull. "American Values and Images: TV Movies and
the First Decade of AIDS." *Journal of Popular Film and Television* 21(1)
(1993): 19-26.

Piontek, Thomas. "Unsafe Representations: Cultural Criticism in the Age of
AIDS." *Discourse* 15(1) (1992): 128-153.

Pryor, John B. and Glenn D. Reeder, Eds. *The Social Psychology of HIV Infection*.
Hillsdale, NJ: Lawrence Erlbaum Associates, 1993.

Riggle, Ellen, Alan L. Ellis, and Anne M. Crawford. "The Impact of 'Media
Contact' on Attitudes Toward Gay Men." *Journal of Homosexuality* 31(3)
(1996): 55-69.

Rogers, Everett and Corinne Shefner-Rogers. "Diffusion of Innovations and HIV/
AIDS Prevention Research." In *Power in the Blood: A Handbook on AIDS,
Politics, and Communication*, Ed. William N. Elwood. Mahwah, NJ: Law-
rence Erlbaum Associates, 1999, pp. 405-414.

Roth, Nancy L. and Linda K. Fuller, Eds. *Women and AIDS: Negotiating Safer Practices, Care, and Representation*. Binghamton, NY: Harrington Park Press, 1998.

Rushing, William A. *The AIDS Epidemic: Social Dimensions of an Infectious Disease*. San Francisco, CA: Westview Press, 1995.

Schatz, Thomas. "The Family Melodrama." *Imitations of Life: A Reader on Film and Television Melodrama*, Ed. Marcia Landy. Detroit, MI: Wayne State University Press, 1991, pp. 148-166.

Seckinger, Beverly and Janet Jakobsen. "Love, Death, and Videotape: *Silverlake Life*." *Between the Sheets, In the Streets: Queer, Lesbian, Gay Documentary*, Eds. Chris Holmlund and Cynthia Fuchs. Minneapolis, MN: University of Minnesota Press, 1997, pp. 144-157.

Shapiro, Benjamin. "Universal Truths: Cultural Myths and Generic Adaptation in 1950s Science Fiction Films." *Journal of Popular Film and Television* 18(3) (1990): 103-111.

Shilts, Randy. *And the Band Played On*. New York: St. Martin's Press, 1987.

Slagle, R. Anthony. "Scapegoating and Political Discourse: Representative Robert Dornan's Legislation of Morality Through HIV/AIDS." In *Power in the Blood: A Handbook on AIDS, Politics, and Communication*, Ed. William N. Elwood. Mahwah, NJ: Lawrence Erlbaum Associates, 1999, pp. 93-104.

Slater, Michael D. "Processing Social Information in Messages: Social Group Familiarity, Fiction Versus Nonfiction, and Subsequent Beliefs." *Communication Research* 17(3) (1990): 327-343.

Sobchack, Thomas. "Genre Film: A Classical Experience." In *Film Genre Reader II*, Ed. Barry Keith Grant. Austin, TX: University of Texas Press, 1995, pp. 102-113.

Sobchack, Vivian. *Screening Space: The American Science Fiction Film*. New York: Ungar, 1997.

Sobnosky, Matthew J. and Eric Hauser. "Initiating or Avoiding Activism: Red Ribbons, Pink Triangles, and Public Argument About AIDS." In *Power in the Blood: A Handbook on AIDS, Politics, and Communication*, Ed. William N. Elwood. Mahwah, NJ: Lawrence Erlbaum Associates, 1999, pp. 25-38.

Sontag, Susan. *Illness As Metaphor and AIDS and Its Metaphors*. New York: Anchor Books, 1989.

Stevens, Sally J. and John G. Bogart. "Reducing HIV Risk Behaviors of Drug-Involved Women: Social, Economic, Medical, and Legal Constraints." In *Power in the Blood: A Handbook on AIDS, Politics, and Communication*, Ed. William N. Elwood. Mahwah, NJ: Lawrence Erlbaum Associates, 1999, pp. 107-120.

Svenkerud, Peer J., Nagesh Rao, and Everett M. Rogers. "Mass Media Effects Through Interpersonal Communication: The Role of 'Twende na Wakati' on the Adoption of HIV/AIDS Prevention in Tanzania." In *Power in the Blood: A Handbook on AIDS, Politics, and Communication*, Ed. William N. Elwood. Mahwah, NJ: Lawrence Erlbaum Associates, 1999, pp. 243-253.

Walters, Timothy N., Lynne M. Walters, and Susanna Hornig Priest. "What We Say and How We Say It: The Influence of Psychosocial Characteristics and

Message Content of HIV/AIDS Public Service Announcements." In *Power in the Blood: A Handbook on AIDS, Politics, and Communication*, Ed. William N. Elwood. Mahwah, NJ: Lawrence Erlbaum Associates, 1999, pp. 293-307.

Watney, Simon. *Policing Desire: Pornography, AIDS and the Media*. Minneapolis, MN: University of Minnesota Press, 1996.

Wheeler, David L. "As AIDS Continues to Spread, Some Scientists Are Pessimistic About Developing a Vaccine." *The Chronicle of Higher Education,* March 26 (1999): A21.

Wimmer, Roger D. and Joseph R. Dominick. *Mass Media Research: An Introduction*. Belmont, CA: Wadsworth Publishing Company, 1991.

Wright, Eric R. "The Social Construction of AIDS." In *Teaching the Sociology of HIV/AIDS*, Eds. Eric R. Wright and Michael Polgar. Washington, DC: ASA Teaching Resources Center, 1997, pp. 69-88.

Yep, Gust A. and Myrna Pietri. "In Their Own Words: Communication and the Politics of HIV Education for Transgenders and Transsexuals in Los Angeles." In *Power in the Blood: A Handbook on AIDS, Politics, and Communication,* Ed. William N. Elwood. Mahwah, NJ: Lawrence Erlbaum Associates, 1999, pp. 199-213.

Zuckerman, Laurence. "Open Season on Gays: AIDS Sparks an Epidemic of Violence Against Homosexuals." *Time,* Vol. 131, No. 10, March 7, 1988: 24.

Zupan, Cheryl. "Clinton Declares AIDS Emergency for Minorities." *Between the Lines,* November 26 (1998): 13.

Index

Activism, 70, 95
Adolescents
    appealing AIDS messages for, 62,
        84
    as characters in AIDS movies,
        62, 63
    as high-risk group members, *ix*,
        5, 60
    and perceived risk of contracting
        HIV/AIDS, 64
Africa, 2, 3, 98
African Americans
    as characters in AIDS movies,
        61, 63, 87, 88
    as high-risk group members, 5, 60,
        61, 64
AIDS
    accepted ways to discuss, 8
    adoption of term, 4, 45
    anal intercourse and, 38, 39
    and the city, 67-76
    and the country, 76-80
    death rate from, 97
    and dementia, 75
    demographics and, 5, 58, 60, 64, 98
    discovery of, 4, 45, 73
    and distancing strategies, 36-37,
        43, 59-60, 65, 87
    future outlook regarding, 12,
        97-98
    as a "gay disease," 3-5, 32, 45-47,
        58, 60, 65, 91
    and heterosexuals, 5, 59
    high-risk behaviors and, 47, 53, 60
    high-risk groups and, 4, 5, 45,
        60, 64
    "invention" of, 6

AIDS *(continued)*
    invincibility and, 3, 64
    long-term consequences of, 4
    rapid spread of, 73-74, 97
    research operationalization of, 9, 48
    retroviruses and, 4
    scapegoating and, 38
    social definition of, 6
    "sufferers," 7
    victim blaming and, 12, 36, 39-43,
        86-90
    victim continuum and, 39-40
    "victims," 7
AIDS metaphor movies, 9, 12, 81,
        87-91, 98
AIDS movies
    absence of cities in, 68
    adolescent central characters
        and, 41-42, 62-63, 76
    African-American central
        characters in, 63
    "AIDS characters" in, 48
    aura of scientific credibility in,
        21-22
    bisexual central characters in, 49
    city as AIDS dystopia in, 67,
        72-76, 80
    city as gay utopia in, 67, 68-72,
        73, 80
    country as balm in, 76-80
    definition of, 9
    eradication of social otherness in,
        29, 30
    female central characters in
        female adolescents as, 40-41,
        62-63, 76

Order Your Own Copy of
This Important Book for Your Personal Library!

THE AIDS MOVIE
Representing a Pandemic in Film and Television

_____ in hardbound at $39.95 (ISBN: 0-7890-1107-7)

_____ in softbound at $17.95 (ISBN: 0-7890-1108-5)

COST OF BOOKS_____	☐ **BILL ME LATER:** ($5 service charge will be added) (Bill-me option is good on US/Canada/Mexico orders only; not good to jobbers, wholesalers, or subscription agencies.)
OUTSIDE USA/CANADA/ MEXICO: ADD 20%_____	
POSTAGE & HANDLING_____ *(US: $4.00 for first book & $1.50 for each additional book Outside US: $5.00 for first book & $2.00 for each additional book)*	☐ Check here if billing address is different from shipping address and attach purchase order and billing address information. Signature_____
SUBTOTAL_____	☐ **PAYMENT ENCLOSED: $**_____
IN CANADA: ADD 7% GST_____	☐ **PLEASE CHARGE TO MY CREDIT CARD.**
STATE TAX_____ *(NY, OH & MN residents, please add appropriate local sales tax)*	☐ Visa ☐ MasterCard ☐ AmEx ☐ Discover ☐ Diner's Club ☐ Eurocard ☐ JCB
FINAL TOTAL_____ *(If paying in Canadian funds, convert using the current exchange rate. UNESCO coupons welcome.)*	Account # _____ Exp. Date _____ Signature _____

Prices in US dollars and subject to change without notice.

NAME _____

INSTITUTION _____

ADDRESS _____

CITY _____

STATE/ZIP _____

COUNTRY _____ COUNTY (NY residents only) _____

TEL _____ FAX _____

E-MAIL_____

May we use your e-mail address for confirmations and other types of information? ☐ Yes ☐ No
We appreciate receiving your e-mail address and fax number. Haworth would like to e-mail or fax special
discount offers to you, as a preferred customer. **We will never share, rent, or exchange your e-mail
address or fax number.** We regard such actions as an invasion of your privacy.

Order From Your Local Bookstore or Directly From
The Haworth Press, Inc.
10 Alice Street, Binghamton, New York 13904-1580 • USA
TELEPHONE: 1-800-HAWORTH (1-800-429-6784) / Outside US/Canada: (607) 722-5857
FAX: 1-800-895-0582 / Outside US/Canada: (607) 772-6362
E-mail: getinfo@haworthpressinc.com
PLEASE PHOTOCOPY THIS FORM FOR YOUR PERSONAL USE.
www.HaworthPress.com

BOF00

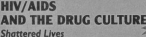